Antiblackness and Global Health

'A compelling account of how antiblackness and colonialism maintain a grip on the epistemic – and, by extension, material – infrastructure of global health, showing us where to aim the hammer in our efforts to knock them off.'
—Seye Abimbola, University of Sydney

'This book reveals the faultlines of inequality and racism in global health formed by colonialism and how they continue to shape global public health practice. It is a powerful and painful reminder that the effects of colonialism are still apparent today. A must-read for those who care about justice and equity in health.'
—Rashida Ferrand, Director, the Health Research Unit Zimbabwe

'Hirsch offers us a compelling and original account linking antiblackness to the spatialisation and coloniality of contemporary global health practice, and the racial politics of care during a public health emergency.'
—Adia Benton, author, *HIV Exceptionalism: Development Through Disease in Sierra Leone*

'In this conceptually ambitious polemic, Hirsch adroitly applies concepts from Black Studies to identify and critique hidden layers of racial bias in epidemic responses. Hirsch's innovative thinking and compassionate narrative make this book essential reading in critical global health studies.'
—Simukai Chigudu, Associate Professor of African Politics, Oxford University

Anthropology, Culture and Society

Series Editors:
Holly High, Deakin University
and
Joshua O. Reno, Binghamton University

Recent titles:

Vicious Games:
Capitalism and Gambling
REBECCA CASSIDY

Anthropologies of Value
EDITED BY LUIS FERNANDO ANGOSTO-
FERRANDEZ AND GEIR HENNING
PRESTERUDSTUEN

Ethnicity and Nationalism:
Anthropological Perspectives
Third Edition
THOMAS HYLLAND ERIKSEN

Small Places, Large Issues:
An Introduction to Social
and Cultural Anthropology
Fifth Edition
THOMAS HYLLAND ERIKSEN

What is Anthropology?
Second Edition
THOMAS HYLLAND ERIKSEN

Anthropology and Development:
Challenges for the Twenty-first Century
KATY GARDNER AND DAVID LEWIS

As If Already Free:
Anthropology and Activism
After David Graeber
EDITED BY HOLLY HIGH
AND JOSHUA O. RENO

Seeing like a Smuggler:
Borders from Below
EDITED BY MAHMOUD KESHAVARZ
AND SHAHRAM KHOSRAVI

How We Struggle:
A Political Anthropology of Labour
SIAN LAZAR

Private Oceans:
The Enclosure and Marketisation
of the Seas
FIONA MCCORMACK

Grassroots Economies:
Living with Austerity in Southern Europe
EDITED BY SUSANA NAROTZKY

Caring Cash:
Free Money and the Ethics
of Solidarity in Kenya
TOM NEUMARK

Rubbish Belongs to the Poor:
Hygienic Enclosure and the
Waste Commons
PATRICK O'HARE

The Rise of Nerd Politics:
Digital Activism and Political Change
JOHN POSTILL

Ground Down by Growth:
Tribe, Caste, Class and Inequality in
Twenty-First-Century India
ALPA SHAH, JENS LERCHE, ET AL

Audit Culture:
How Indicators and Rankings are
Reshaping the World
CRIS SHORE AND SUSAN WRIGHT

The Paradox of Svalbard:
Climate Change and Globalisation
in the Arctic
ZDENKA SOKOLÍČKOVÁ

Watershed Politics and Climate Change
in Peru
ASTRID B. STENSRUD

When Protest Becomes Crime:
Politics and Law in Liberal Democracies
CAROLIJN TERWINDT

Antiblackness and Global Health

A Response to Ebola in the Colonial Wake

Lioba Hirsch

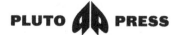

First published 2024 by Pluto Press
New Wing, Somerset House, Strand, London WC2R 1LA
and Pluto Press, Inc.
1930 Village Center Circle, 3-834, Las Vegas, NV 89134

www.plutobooks.com

British Library Cataloguing in Publication Data
A catalogue record for this book is available from the British Library

ISBN 978 0 7453 4628 1 Paperback
ISBN 978 0 7453 4632 8 PDF
ISBN 978 0 7453 4630 4 EPUB

This book is printed on paper suitable for recycling and made from fully
managed and sustained forest sources. Logging, pulping and manufacturing
processes are expected to conform to the environmental standards of the
country of origin.

Typeset by Stanford DTP Services, Northampton, England

Simultaneously printed in the United Kingdom and United States of America

You see, it's not just an intellectual struggle. [...] It was an understanding that, as Lewis Gordon has been the first to keep insisting, we live in an anti-Black world – a systemically anti-Black world; and therefore whites are not [simply] 'racists'. They too live in the same world in which we live. The truth that structures their minds, their 'consciousness', structures ours.

Sylvia Wynter

I belong to a legacy of those who saw what this world had to offer and refused it. Before they refused it, they fought it, and not just with words. This method emerges from the substance of everyday things. So, *excuse me* if it seems at times like I am grasping at nothing. I am. Hold on with me.

Lola Olufemi

Contents

List of Figures   viii
Series Preface   ix
Acknowledgements   x
Abbreviations   xii
Prologue   xiii

Introduction: Thinking Towards Black Humanity in Global Health   1

1 Place, *Weather* and Disease Control in (Post)Colonial Freetown   19

2 Colonial Mobilities and Infrastructures: The Production of
   (Anti)Blackness   58

3 Thinking and Practising Care: Space, Risk and Racialisation
   in Ebola Treatment Centres   91

4 Wakefulness: Epistemic Spaces, Flows and Epigrammatic
   Antiblackness   123

5 Thinking Global Health Otherwise   156

List of Interviewees   159
Notes   160
References   164
Archival Sources   175
Index   177

Figures

1. Map of Pademba Road Cemetery, bleached by the sun   xvi
2. A section of Pademba Road Cemetery in Waterloo   xvii
3. Sign indicating a safe parking spot in Kent, a village on the
    Freetown Peninsula   21
4. Wilberforce Street in Freetown   25
5. Excerpt of Freetown map 1913   28
6. Example of British colonial architecture in Hill Station,
    Freetown in 1871 and 2019   29
7. Original plaque on top of King's Yard Gate   37
8. Connaught Hospital and King's Yard Gate   37
9. Old landing dock, Bunce Island, Sierra Leone   64
10. Imperial Airways October 1931 'Empire' routes   68
11. Map of Ebola treatment centre drawn from memory by Dina   105

Series Preface

As people around the world confront the inequality and injustice of new forms of oppression, as well as the impacts of human life on planetary ecosystems, this book series asks what anthropology can contribute to the crises and challenges of the twenty-first century. Our goal is to establish a distinctive anthropological contribution to debates and discussions that are often dominated by politics and economics. What is sorely lacking, and what anthropological methods can provide, is an appreciation of the human condition.

We publish works that draw inspiration from traditions of ethnographic research and anthropological analysis to address power and social change while keeping the struggles and stories of human beings centre stage. We welcome books that set out to make anthropology matter, bringing classic anthropological concerns with exchange, difference, belief, kinship and the material world into engagement with contemporary environmental change, capitalist economy and forms of inequality. We publish work from all traditions of anthropology, combining theoretical debate with empirical evidence to demonstrate the unique contribution anthropology can make to understanding the contemporary world.

Holly High and Joshua O. Reno

Acknowledgements

This is a book for health justice. It is for all those and thanks to all those who work to build solidarities and who do the physical and intellectual work of dismantling unjust and oppressive systems anywhere. May you remain hopeful and angry. We are many.

For my mother, who taught me to listen with care, and my father who is teaching me to fight. For Christina, who is teaching me patience. To Louisa and Leander. And Uta.

This book would not exist without everyone who gifted me their time and shared their experiences, at times painful and difficult, at times joyful. Thank you for trusting me with these bits of your worlds, thank you for laughing and crying with me. Thank you to the healthcare workers of Salone and to all those fighting for health justice in West Africa. To Mohamed Barrie without whom none of my research in Sierra Leone would have happened. To the Sierra Leone Urban Research Centre, my first academic home in Freetown. To everyone in the Sierra Leonean diaspora in the UK, in Germany and Switzerland: thank you.

A special thanks to Mateusz Zatonski for his kindness, intellectual curiosity and generous spirit.

Work that went into this book was funded by a Heinrich-Böll Foundation PhD scholarship from 2015 to 2018 and a UCL (University College London) cross-disciplinary training scholarship from 2018 to 2019. I finished writing this book while being funded by a Wellcome Research Fellowship in Humanities and Social Sciences.

To everyone at Pluto Press, thank you for taking this project on, especially David Castle, and the entire editorial, production and marketing teams: Robert Webb, Emily Orford, Jonila Krasniqi, Sophie O'Reirdan, Patrick Hughes. And a huge thanks to Sophie Richmond for copy-editing.

Thank you to Professor Alan Ingram, who supervised this work when it was still struggling to become a PhD thesis, who was patient and rigorous and encouraged my intellectual curiosity. Also, to Professor Ben Page for his guidance and generosity. To my generous and brilliant PhD examiners Professor Patricia Noxolo and Dr Caroline Bressey: we need more academics like you. This book is also the product of important friendships that emerged out of pursuing PhDs in UCL's Department of Geography and Institute for Global Health: thanks to Sarah Kunz, Lo Marshall, Tania Guerrero, Niranjana, Clement Oghoro, Laura Cuch, Hui-Chun Liu, Gümeç Karamak, Nathaniel Telemaque, Sarah Amele and Sandra Iheanacho. Also and especially to Jamie Schaerer and Ruba Huleihel. Thank you for your friendships, they sustain me.

I worked at three different institutions and on three different research projects while this book very slowly came into being. Thank you to colleagues at LSHTM (the London School of Hygiene and Tropical Medicine), especially John Manton, Coll de Lima Hutchison, Pippa Grenfell, Emilie Koum Besson, Mishal Khan, Martin Gorsky and Ingrid James. At the University of Liverpool: to Ruth Cheung-Judge and Shelda-Jane Smith. Also, Bethan Evans and Kathy Burrell. At the University of Edinburgh: Chisomo Kalinga and especially Jamie Cross and Alice Street for thinking that this work had the potential to be a book in the first place. To Alice, again, for mentoring me and continuously believing in my work.

And to Myfanwy James, Eleanor Davies and Molly Naisanga and Adia Benton, Seye Abimbola and James Smith. Everyone here, even if you were unaware of it, helped shaped my thinking and writing while I wrote this book.

To Aidan: for everything here and everything else. Und für Ama. Sei unerschrocken und frei.

Abbreviations

AIDS – acquired immunodeficiency syndrome
BIPOC – Black, Indigenous and other People of Colour
CDC – Centers for Disease Control
DFID – Department for International Development
DRC – Democratic Republic of Congo
EDI – Equality, Diversity and Inclusion
EHU – Ebola holding unit
ETC – Ebola treatment centre
EVD – Ebola virus disease
HIV – human immunodeficiency virus
IMATT – International Military Advisory and Training Team
IPC – infection prevention and control
MSF – Médecins sans Frontières/Doctors without Borders
NGO – non-governmental organisation
NHS – National Health Service (UK)
PHE – Public Health England
PPE – personal protective equipment
WHO – World Health Organization

Prologue

2007

I have suffered from atopic dermatitis since I was a baby. The doctors told my parents that the condition, which can make patches of the skin feel like they have become paper thin and rough or look like they are inflamed, scaly and wet, but which are always, always intensely itchy and lead to the unbearable urge to scratch, is caused by environmental factors, in particular stress and anxiety. So it seems that I was born anxious and that my skin has always, at least in part, reflected my relation to the world and my anxiety, even before I was able to walk and talk and articulate my feelings and worries. There is no cure for atopic dermatitis and my mother refused the application of cortisone. I lived with atopic dermatitis until I was about four or five. Then the symptoms stopped and I stopped scratching my skin every night.

However, symptoms of atopic dermatitis can come and go. They can vanish and then reoccur again after several years. I remained itch-free through most of my childhood and early teenage years until I left home to go to school in France for a year at the age of 16. It was difficult finding a host family for me; I was told by someone at the agency that people didn't want a Black teenager. They preferred more 'typical' white German girls. France was fine. I relished my increased sense of independence and being able to speak French, one of the languages spoken by my father's family in Togo. I returned to Berlin a year later, a patch of skin on my shin, itchy and scaly, inflamed and oozing. I don't blame France for this, it just happened. I was still anxious, and especially about the appearance of my skin, but also a teenager and somewhat carefree. My experience of primary health care had been good so far, I didn't know yet all the forms that antiblack racism can take. I still don't. To this date, it still sometimes takes me a while to process racism. I check in with myself and take stock: 'Yes, that was racist', I will think a day later. Although my brain affords me these brief reprieves, this privileged ignorance occurs less and less often the older I become. The protective shield of Black friendships and love and knowledge that my mother built around me – a shield that felt both physical and epistemic and emotional – grows thinner every day, like my skin.

I was not seen by my usual GP when I went to the surgery to have someone look at my leg. I hadn't had symptoms of atopic dermatitis in years and this one, I admit, looked different: angry and red and scaly. It had never looked that way before. So, it is possible that I didn't say to the doctor that this might be atopic dermatitis, that I simply presented myself to the office to which I had been coming since I was a child to seek health advice and care. My regular GP – the one who had treated me since I was a child – was not in. It was the summer and maybe he was on annual leave or he just wasn't working that day. The doctor who was in seemed young, although that is no excuse; it is simply the only thing I remember. That and that he had black hair. He looked at my leg and looked at me and typed some notes on his computer. I don't remember much else. Maybe he made me get up on the examination table, maybe he simply came around his desk and looked at my leg with me in the chair, sitting there, telling him about this patch of skin that was itchy and uncomfortable and also (I was 17) did not look good.

I remember him sitting behind his desk and asking me if it could be AIDS (acquired immunodeficiency syndrome). I think I just laughed. To my teenage self that seemed incredibly unlikely – because it was. I remember him stating it, more firmly this time, maybe as a reaction to my laughter (did I not take the situation seriously?): 'This could be AIDS.'

I don't remember much else after that, but I remember not feeling particularly worried. Maybe that protective shield still worked and logic prevailed. Maybe, being 17 and filled with teenage confidence, there was very little that could have burst my bubble. Maybe I was laughing to protect myself, to distance myself from a diagnosis that could change my life forever. I don't know. Maybe the way in which he delivered his diagnosis seemed to me, even then, careless, rather than authoritative. Maybe I remembered my long, yet distant history of atopic dermatitis and the fact that my medical history was right there for him to read on his computer, the computer he was typing on; that it was there with us, in this office to which I had come to be examined for this very disease so often when I was a small child. In any case, I remember not leaving that doctor's office feeling fearful.

I am also not sure when it dawned on me that what had just happened was bad, careless and racist; that it should not have happened; that you should never diagnose a young person with a serious, potentially life-altering disease, without an adult present and based on a mere glance at their skin. That you should do blood tests and get a second opinion at the very least and ask that person to come back, with a parent, once you were sure. Maybe I realised all this when calling my mother on the way home, on a sunny S-Bahn platform, waiting for the next train and acutely aware that people nearby might overhear, but also unable to wait until I was home to tell her. She exploded, her voice becoming as angry as the skin on my leg. Maybe that reassured me? That I wasn't the only one not believing that I had AIDS. Only later did the full realisation come that my young Black body may have swayed him and provoked that carelessness in him. That he may have seen me and seen my leg and thought: 'AIDS'. That my Black skin colour overshadowed his medical training and duty of care and made him disregard or not bother looking at the file containing my medical history. Or maybe he did look and still thought that the skin on my leg looked like Kaposi's Sarcoma. If he did, he never followed up. I still wonder, if I had been that typical white German girl, would this have happened?

I wonder where that doctor is today, 15 years later, and whether he still carelessly diagnoses young Black women with AIDS.

2019

The Ebola cemetery in Waterloo is located in an overgrown field, less than 5 kilometres from the main road connecting Waterloo and Freetown, Sierra Leone's capital. There are segregated sections, demarcated by cement pillars, each bearing a letter. We walk past sections E, F, J, L and K, each of which contains rows and rows of identical cement headstones, inscribed with the words 'In loving memory of' followed by a name, a burial date, the age of the deceased and a cemetery reference number. In many cases the name of the deceased is unknown and the graves are marked with the phrase 'Known unto God'. Funded through official UK development assistance, Concern Worldwide, an international NGO (non-governmental organisation) in charge of burials at the cemetery, put up signs showing the layout of the cemetery and of individual sections. These signs are bleached by the sun and barely legible. I can hardly make out the official name of the cemetery, 'Paloko Road Cemetery, Waterloo' at the top and, more clearly visible, a British flag over the words 'UK aid' in the lower right-hand corner (Figure 1). The rows and rows of reference numbers, corresponding to the graves on the cemetery, are illegible. The flag and logo are still visible because they alone were printed in colour, the logo mirroring the blue and red of the British flag. The blue metal frame has begun to rust and reddish-brown streaks of colour have bled onto the sign. A thin layer of dust has settled on it and someone (a visitor?) has run their fingers through it, making lines and a star-like shape at the bottom, next to the 'UK aid' logo, which has been wiped clean of dust. Without any protection from the sun and rain the sign will soon be completely illegible. No doubt the Union Jack and 'UK aid' will be the last things that remain.

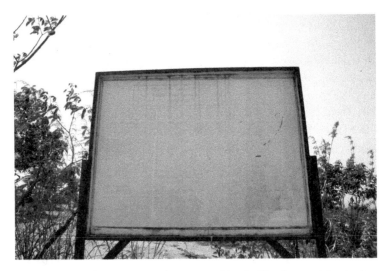

Figure 1   Map of Pademba Road Cemetery, bleached by the sun. The sign is barely legible. (Photo by the author)

Like the sign, the cemetery has become almost invisible. We approach it from the back and are directed to a large, seemingly wild, field. All I can see is tall meadow grass and hedges and trees, growing so closely together that they obscure what lies behind it from view. Two soldiers in civilian clothing tell me to watch for uneven ground as they lead us through the thicket. There is no clear path and, until I see the headstones, I am unaware that the cemetery is right here. Here, on the edge, the grass is taller than me. Thin, light brown plant stalks and low trees make it almost impossible to make out the gravestones. To our left, dry tall grass has taken over and it is impossible to walk between the headstones. To our right a field opens up, similarly overgrown, but with shorter plants: brown stalks crowned with white, pillowy heads. They remind me strongly of cotton; as if these graves might in fact have been dug in a cotton field across the ocean, a cotton field interspersed with light grey uniform headstones for the millions of

Africans who were forcibly enslaved and transported across the Atlantic to work on cotton fields and rice and sugarcane plantations rather than for the thousands of people who died from Ebola in Sierra Leone. The fleeting thought is a reminder of the antiblack violence that has shaped lives on both sides of the Atlantic.

The violence of the Ebola epidemic and the centuries old antiblack violence that characterises enslavement and colonialism in Sierra Leone appear to me, on this meadow, in muted form. The gravestones are visible, yet obscured by the cotton-like plants, which have grown tall and dense in places, making it more difficult to make out names and dates (Figure 2). At the same time, the plant growing here is not cotton, and a closer look confirms this; but the association with cotton is strong, so strong that one of my companions notices it too. A cotton field does not automatically conjure the transatlantic slave trade. In this particular location, however, and for me, a Black researcher, having conducted months of research on antiblackness and Ebola virus disease, it is reminiscent of Sierra Leone's long, forced integration into the transatlantic world through the slave trade and British colonialism. In this cemetery, as in my research, antiblackness often underlies what is immediately tangible. The rows of graves, holding hundreds of bodies, are more tangible than the cotton-like plants. Yet, to me, in this

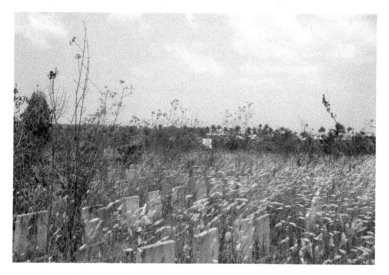

Figure 2   A section of Pademba Road Cemetery in Waterloo. The graves are all of people who died during the Sierra Leonean Ebola epidemic. (Photo by the author)

place, both evoke Black death and antiblack violence. At times this anti-blackness takes careful work to discern or prior knowledge to understand. In my research, as in the cemetery, I actively foreground antiblackness through associations; I infer it from silences and trace its marginalisations.

In the Ebola cemetery in Waterloo, the faded sign, the still colourful Union Jack and the cotton-like plants between rows of headstones are evocative of the themes and methods I explore and draw on in this book. They suggest that landscapes contain the possibility of multiple realities, of layered histories and geographies. If we explore such associations and connections further, we can also detect the persistence of antiblackness and the ambiguous nature of British involvement in relation to the Ebola epidemic in Sierra Leone. Doing so requires a researcher to be aware of the ways in which legacies of colonialism and the slave trade continue to hold Black life in the present.[1] They also signal the non-linear methodology that I adopted in conducting the research, warranted by the marginalisation and elusiveness of antiblackness in the colonial present.

I start *Antiblackness and Global Health* with an account of these two experiences, twelve years apart and taking place in different parts of the world, for two reasons: On the one hand, they allow me to place myself in this research and analysis as an active participant, rather than a disembodied voice. Such a positioning, I argue, is honest and necessary. On the other hand, both accounts are symptomatic of antiblackness in health; of the intimate, personal, political and systematic ways in which antiblackness shapes and intrudes in health management on the individual and global level and the sometimes clear, sometimes unfocused ways in which we discern it. These two accounts also spell out an important truth about anti-blackness and antiblack racism: like Blackness, experiences of antiblack racism and systemic antiblackness are always felt and embodied. Another researcher or person might not see what I see or might draw different conclusions. Therein lies the difficulty of translating antiblackness epis-temically. The genius of white supremacy and a side-product of living in a world that is still dominated by whiteness is that it leaves you with a con-stant feeling of not being quite sure, a niggling sense of doubt, an anxiety, an epistemic hierarchy that discounts Black experiences as unscientific and places them at the bottom. *I know antiblackness, but how can I be sure? The doctor may not have been racist at all. This plant looks nothing like cotton.* This sense of doubt is made worse when working in the fields of global health and medicine. Medicine, we are assured, is objective, impartial and apolitical. Skin colour has no bearing on the inner workings of the human body and so medicine and medical practice are removed from dealing with discrimination and inequality. In medicine the intimate and the political are often separate. In Black Studies and postcolonial theory, and in our lives and bodies, they are deeply entangled. This book deals with the entanglements, the 'condition of being twisted together or entwined [...] even if it was resisted, or ignored or uninvited' (Nuttall, 2009) of antiblackness and global health. These entanglements are necessarily present, if we accept that we live, as Sylvia Wynter put it, in an antiblack world. That we live, to use Christina Sharpe's powerful concept, 'in the wake', the aftermath of enslavement and colonialism. An aftermath that overtakes history to reach into the present. Sharpe (2016, p. 104) writes: 'In my text, the weather is the totality of our environments; the weather is the total climate; and that climate is antiblack.' That antiblackness is real and a constitutive aspect of our modernity is thus the premise on which this book is based. How antiblackness manifests in global health, is its topic.

Introduction: Thinking Towards Black Humanity in Global Health

This is a retelling of constellations.[1]

Sierra Leone's leading haemorrhagic fever specialist had tested positive for Ebola virus disease on 22 July after treating patients with Ebola at Kenema Government Hospital, in the eastern part of the country. As a virologist, and having been in charge of the country's Lassa fever programme, Dr Khan was aware of the risks of treating infectious haemorrhagic fevers. According to reports and interviews with him and his colleagues before and after his passing he was meticulous about donning protective gear before attending to patients. To reassure patients and fight the stigma, he made a habit of hugging those who had recovered from Ebola upon being discharged from the hospital. Nevertheless, he and several nurses at the Kenema hospital contracted the virus. So as not to be treated by his own colleagues, Dr Khan was transported to Kailahun, a town close to the Guinean border to an MSF (Doctors without Borders) treatment facility. His condition seemed to improve before worsening (*The New Humanitarian*, 2014).

A month earlier, scientists from the Public Health Agency of Canada who had been instrumental in co-developing ZMapp, Mapp Pharmaceuticals' experimental Ebola drug, travelled to Kailahun with three doses of ZMapp. They left at least one of these doses in a freezer in MSF's newly established Ebola treatment centre in Kailahun, allegedly to test how ZMapp would hold up in a field hospital in the hot climate (Thomas, 2019a).

Meanwhile at Dr Khan's bedside, MSF and WHO (World Health Organization) doctors are debating what to do. They know of the one dose of ZMapp available to them and have been authorised to use it to try to cure Dr Khan. But they're unsure. His blood results show Ebola antibodies, a sign that his body has begun to fight the disease on its own. ZMapp has never been tested on humans before. What if it interferes with his body's immune system? What if he dies not of Ebola but of the drug? They worry too that Dr Khan's death as a result of the experimental use of ZMapp will interfere with their general public health response. 'What they really didn't want to do was kill Dr Khan with their attempt at therapy. If word got out that MSF killed Dr Khan, that would have implications for outbreak control,' Armand Sprecher, one of MSF's public health specialists would later say to the *New York Times* (Pollack, 2014). Dr Khan is still showing relatively mild symptoms of the disease. He does not yet have diarrhoea or vomiting, is alert and conscious, and is meant to be moved to a European hospital shortly. Maybe it would be better to administer the ZMapp there, in a more controlled environment? They don't come to a unanimous decision, and they don't consult Dr Khan or his family either, the reasoning being that it would be unethical to propose treatment only to withdraw it later. They also have concerns about singling out Dr Khan for treatment because he is a famous virologist and some members of staff threaten to resign should he be offered the drug (O'Dempsey, 2017). The MSF team decide not to try the ZMapp on Dr Khan. Dr Khan's condition deteriorates, he starts having diarrhoea and vomiting and the company charged with evacuating him, International SOS, refuses to take him. He dies on 29 July in Kailahun.

Meanwhile, in neighbouring Liberia, two Americans have also contracted Ebola. Both work for Samaritan's Purse, a Christian medical mission, in an Ebola treatment centre, one as a doctor, one as a nurse. Their doctors are aware of that dose of ZMapp only a few hundred kilometres away in Kailahun. As in Dr Khan's case, the doctors in charge of the Americans' care debate whether they should use ZMapp to try to cure them. They consult the patients themselves, who agree to the experimental treatment. A CDC (Centers for Disease Control) official in Monrovia flies to Kailahun to retrieve the drug on 29 July (Thomas, 2019a). At least one of them is treated with ZMapp before they are evacuated to Atlanta to receive further treatment. Both survive.

Different medical teams are in charge of the American health workers and Dr Khan, and their decision-making processes play out independently from one another. Nevertheless, the cases are linked by that one dose of ZMapp. In this constellation, the decision to withhold the experimental drug from the Sierra Leonean doctor enables the treatment of the Americans. The *New York Times* (Pollack, 2014) article which reported the doctors' decision not to use ZMapp on Dr Khan homed in on 'the already fragile public trust in international efforts to contain the world's worst Ebola outbreak'. This is put forward as a reason to deny Dr Khan the experimental treatment with ZMapp. The fact that this fragile public trust was itself a consequence of layered histories of colonial and postcolonial abuses of power, often in conjunction with medical care and research, seems to have exceeded the realms of the article's analysis. The lack of public trust in international health responses, according to the article, had no bearing on the privileged access to the drug the American doctors received, nor it seems, did the optics of treating them, rather than Liberian patients in the same treatment centre.

The next constellation is more straightforward.

Dr Olivet Buck contracted Ebola in early September 2014.[2] She had been caring for patients at Lumley Government Hospital in Freetown, Sierra Leone's capital. Dr Buck was the fourth Sierra Leonean doctor to contract Ebola after treating affected patients in just a few months. In an effort to save her life, Sierra Leonean president Ernest Bai Koroma appealed to the WHO to airlift her to Germany for treatment. The WHO refused. Dr Buck died late on Saturday 13 September 2014 in Sierra Leone.

Meanwhile, Dutch officials were preparing the evacuation of two Dutch doctors who had come into direct, unprotected contact with a patient who subsequently died of Ebola at the Dutch-run Lion Heart Medical Centre in Yele in Sierra Leone's Tonkolili District. The doctors fled to the nearest Dutch embassy in Ghana from where they were medevac'd by International SOS. At the point of evacuation both doctors were asymptomatic. Neither fell ill after the exposure (Reuters Staff, 2014).

As with the case of Dr Khan and the American doctors, what is at stake here is the question of Black/African agency. When analysed alongside the treatment, evacuation and survival of the two missionaries at Samaritan's Purse, Dr Khan's death showcases the deliberate stripping away of his agency both as a medical professional and as a patient. In this context, it seems, medical humanitarianism treats Black bodies, not people (let alone qualified virologists). In the case of Dr Olivet Buck, the WHO's refusal to medevac her to a hospital in which she could receive better treatment speaks of institutional short-sightedness and the refusal to see the survival of a Sierra Leonean doctor as an important resource in the Sierra Leonean fight against Ebola. Had she survived her body would have presented antibodies, making it safer for her to keep working with Ebola patients. In conjunction with the actions of the two Dutch doctors however, Dr Buck's case also speaks to something else: to an unequal treatment regime and the humanitarian *politics of life* (Fassin, 2007), to the differentiation between lives to be saved and lives to be risked. Due to the continued colonial power dynamics of humanitarianism – of who intervenes in the lives of whom – white lives are usually saved. Black lives, it often seems, are expendable. However rather than only reading this as a feature of humanitarian work, Black Studies points to the foundational nature of this expendability. The Black exclusion from humanity, or from forms of humanity worthy of being saved, is constitutive of our modernity (Wynter, 2003; Weheliye, 2015). Weheliye argues in *Habeas Viscus* (2015, p. 50) that 'race is not a biological category that is politically charged. It is a political category that has been disguised as a biological one.' In global health interventions, this conflation is further amplified and obscured.

Amidst the violence and deaths of the Ebola outbreak in West Africa, I am not the first one to put these four incidents in constellation with one another. However, I draw them out specifically because they foreshadow antiblack undercurrents in global health management generally and in the Sierra Leonean Ebola epidemic of 2014–16 in particular. WHO is subject to 'institutional rigidity' (O'Dempsey, 2017), as was the case with MSF's refusal to administer ZMapp to Dr Khan or 'bureaucratic red tape' (Benton, 2014), which prevented the evacuation of Dr Buck to a hospital in Germany, and who is not, clearly played out along antiblack lines. Or, to put it differently, whose lives the international community could save and whose lives it proved too difficult, too costly or unethical to save, was, at least to a certain extent and as this constellation of cases shows, linked to a patient's country of birth, but was made visible through the colour of their skin and their degree of *locality*. The removal of Black African agency and deliberate stripping of capacity for self-help, we have come to learn, often become by-products of international efforts to contain crises and emergencies, even when they are ostensibly designed to prevent exactly that.

This book works by foregrounding such constellations. Not to point the finger of blame at any one individual or organisation, but to unearth the antiblack fault-lines on which global health is built and which play out painfully in contemporary global health emergencies and their management. To some of us, these have been painfully obvious all along. For others they are barely visible. The cost of leaving these currents untouched, of engaging in the privilege of 'denying constellational thinking' (Cole, 2012), lies in the loss of Black lives and Black agency on the African continent and elsewhere. To borrow a phrase of Teju Cole's (2012) writing on the white saviour industrial complex: 'If we are going to interfere in the lives of others, a little due diligence is the minimum requirement.' *Antiblackness and Global Health* centres care for Black life and a recognition of the pervasiveness of colonial antiblackness in, and in relation to, Sierra Leone in its critical analyses of the British-led international response to the 2014–16 Ebola epidemic in that country. This analysis of a specific global health event allows the book to make three conceptual contributions, which speak to antiblackness in global health more generally: First, it analyses the Ebola response through the lens of Black Studies in order to foreground antiblack constellations. Second, and building on this first analytical intervention, it showcases how Black Studies can contribute critical insights into the study of global health in and, to a certain extent, beyond Sierra Leone. Third, the book removes Black Studies from its traditional geographical remit, the Americas, to put forward the concept of *colonial antiblackness*, a framework to understand how antiblackness plays out in the aftermath of colonialism in, and in relation to, sub-Saharan Africa.

Thinking Through Colonial Ruins

In Sierra Leone, infectious disease control was historically bound up with the transatlantic slave trade, the British resettlement of freed slaves in the eighteenth and nineteenth centuries and the subsequent colonisation of Sierra Leone by the British Crown. These historic entanglements resurface, I argue, albeit in elusive, at times ambiguous ways, during the 2014–16 response. They don't always take as explicit a form as in the deaths of Dr Khan and Dr Buck, but their elusiveness means they continue to be left unexamined and contribute to ongoing processes of ruination (Stoler, 2013). *Antiblackness and Global Health* excavates these entanglements by analytically 'placing' the Ebola response in Sierra Leone in the wake of colonialism; that is to say, it considers the response *in* and *as part of* the aftermath of the antiblack violence that has shaped Sierra Leone historically and geographically. This 'placing' is done in two main ways. First, relying on research conducted in British archives of colonial disease control and research in Sierra Leone, I analyse the international Ebola response with reference to historical infrastructures, landscapes, epistemologies and practices that are suffused by antiblackness and which underlie present-day infectious disease control in Sierra Leone. I consider the international Ebola response in the midst of these material and epistemic traces and examine to what extent the antiblack violence that characterises this past resurfaces around the response. By considering the past and present of antiblack violence in relation to infectious disease control in Sierra Leone, this placing questions the temporal linearity which constitutes one aspect of postcolonialism. It also opens up the possibility of 'different geographic stories' (McKittrick, 2006, p. x), stories in which the past and present coexist geographically. Second, relying on in-depth interviews with international health responders and members of the Sierra Leonean diaspora, I trace the discursive continuities, marginalisations and silences that acknowledge or deny antiblack entanglements in narrations of the 2014–16 response. This second 'placing' takes the form of unpacking absences and locating the colonial wake spatially and discursively. I present an account of the Ebola epidemic that foregrounds the echoes, resonances and associations between the colonial past and the 2014–16 British-led international Ebola response. Overall, the book shows that approaching the wake of colonialism and questions of health and disease through each other allows us to rethink how and where we study colonial antiblackness in the present. Here, colonial health management is not studied as a past phenomenon, but as shaping Black ontology in the present. Simultaneously, *Antiblackness and Global Health* argues for an understanding of present-day antiblackness that exceeds police violence and the prison-industrial complex, and includes aspects of health and health care provision as a field in which Black ontology is negotiated and contested. There is sorrow here, but there is also joy in resistance and the affirmation of Black and African agency.

Building on an exploration of these historic-contemporary entanglements, I show that colonial antiblackness constitutes a geographical and epistemic reality, which has shaped Sierra Leone in the past and continues to shape it in the present. I demonstrate that this antiblack reality has been largely normalised within Sierra Leone's postcolonial landscape. Furthermore, as the book shows, (colonial) antiblackness was given little consideration in the international Ebola response in Sierra Leone. Indeed, the extent to which antiblackness was normalised became evident in my research: if one looks closely, traces of enslavement and colonialism are readily apparent in Freetown's built environment, in its toponomy and architecture. At the same time, acknowledgement of or reference to this reality was largely absent in responders' narrations of the epidemic. I argue that this disconnect between physical reality and individual sense-making evokes the colonial wake. It also elicits a normalisation of the antiblack violence that has structured how the UK has related to Sierra Leone and that has shaped Black life – and health – in Sierra Leone.

Analysing the 2014–16 Sierra Leonean Ebola outbreak through this lens, one which foregrounds historical entanglements of antiblackness and colonial healthcare, shapes how I approach the definition of a global health event. Following Adia Benton's (2015) work on HIV (human immunodeficiency virus) exceptionalism in Sierra Leone, I analyse the response to the 2014–16 outbreak across different scales. A global health event, in my reading, is never contained geographically or temporally, but is made by the socio-political, economic and historical relations which shape the landscape in which it occurs. The Ebola outbreak and the response which sought to curtail it, become constituted by and build on layers of history and socio-economic and epistemic interactions. Nonetheless, I pay particular attention to the framing of the outbreak as a global health event on a global scale, which stands in contrast to the regional nature of the epidemic. As Alex Nading (2017) has shown, attention needs to be paid to what constitutes a global health event, and to who has the power to define it. This power of definition, I would argue in the case of the British-led international response to the Sierra Leonean Ebola outbreak, was deeply entangled with antiblack sentiments which have shaped how West Africa has been thought of from a European colonial-humanitarian perspective for some time.

This is necessarily an incomplete account and one which tells one amidst a myriad of stories. Which stories of the outbreak and response have been privileged in critical analyses so far, and which ones have been neglected or sidelined is as much subject to colonial dynamics as the events they are recounting themselves. All shortcomings evidenced here are my own. I wrote this book with humility and I hope that it is received as such, even though that does not exempt it, or me, from well-founded critiques. I would like to address two of these first-hand, although there are undoubtedly many more.

In conversations with African scientists and researchers, indeed in conversations with family members and friends, my continued insistence on reading Africa's present through its colonial past often provokes feelings of exasperation. What is the purpose of repeatedly pointing to Black/African victimisation in the past and present? Does my analysis not perpetuate what it accuses the international response of? Namely, the removal of Black/African agency at individual, societal and government levels? Does my analysis let African governments off the hook? All of these are valid questions and I do not think that I can relinquish the responsibility of my work being read in this way. Black Studies, and afro-pessimism as one of its intellectual branches, focuses on antiblackness and antiblack violence, rather than Black and African joy, which are undoubtedly more worthy topics of analysis. However, this is an account of the international response to the Sierra Leonean Ebola outbreak and in my analysis I draw on research conducted with international responders, rather than Sierra Leoneans. I did this not to privilege one account over another, but because I found it necessary to research and publish on the antiblack undercurrents that present a narrative which strips Black Africans of agency and justifies the need for outside humanitarian intervention. I stand by that choice. However, I also acknowledge that it is an imperfect choice and possibly one influenced by my positioning in the diaspora. Since I started working on this book, first as a PhD and then as a manuscript, my thinking has somewhat shifted and evolved. I still love Christina Sharpe's (2016) *In the Wake* for what it taught me and for the care it expresses towards Black life and death. But I have also come to learn to resist the temptation of afro-pessimism as a genre. Our lives are manifold and pluriversal and beautiful, and exceed a reduction to enslavement and antiblackness. Yet, antiblackness undoubtedly persists and shapes our present and our futures. There is tension here and duality. Let's sit with it.

A second flaw in the design of my research is also deeply entangled with British colonialism in Sierra Leone. In my analysis I relied on interviews with international responders who predominantly worked in and around Freetown. Although I included the accounts of Sierra Leonean and international responders who worked in other parts of the country, my analysis is geographically skewed towards Freetown and the Freetown Peninsula. This bias reproduces that of a long line of colonial and postcolonial governments, which have privileged Freetown over the provinces both in terms of financial power and decision making. Many would argue that the civil war only started to be taken seriously once it reached Freetown. Many would argue that the same needs to be said for the Sierra Leonean and international Ebola response. I cannot correct the design flaws inherent in my research, which was conducted between 2016 and 2019. But I do acknowledge that they contribute to a canon of research that has privileged Freetown and Western Area (the administrative region encompassing Freetown and the Freetown Peninsula) more broadly over other parts of Sierra Leone. This bias needs to be at least in part, linked to the progress of British colonialism in Sierra Leone, which focused on Freetown first, before progressively incorporating other parts of Sierra Leone, without, however, ever according the same political and financial investments to those areas. During colonial times, this decision, was also linked to the preponderance of white colonial officers, their families and Krio families in and around Freetown in comparison to eastern, central and northern Sierra Leone.

What is Antiblackness?

The question of the human and the social, of what it means to be human, are central to the humanities and social sciences. At the heart of both disciplinary fields lies the idea of the universality of our humanity, an idea as Costa Vargas and Jung (2021) argue, belied by histories of antiblackness. Indeed, as Sylvia Wynter, Orlando Patterson, Rinaldo Walcott, Alexander Weheliye, Saidiya Hartman, Hortense Spillers and other Black Studies writers have shown, the human, has long been defined *against* the category of Blackness; Black/African people have long been excluded from the category of human. In the Americas, enslavement and antiblack violence have excluded Blackness from the realm of the social and made it congruent with social death (Patterson, 1982). This exclusion, which has deep historical roots, is most closely tied to the enslavement, sale and colonial subjectification of Black Africans. In fact, Sylvia Wynter (1994) dates this exclusion to 1492. It takes one of its earliest forms in the Valladolid debate between Bartolomé de las Casas and Juàn Ginés de Sepúlveda on the subject of the humanity of Native peoples in the Americas in 1550. De las Casas famously argued for the inclusion of Native Americans in the category of humans and against their continued enslavement, whereas Sepúlveda argued against it. To remedy the projected shortfall in labour, de las Casas argued in favour of the enslavement and attendant exclusion from humanity of Black Africans, although he changed his stance later in life. Black Studies, in its modern interpretation, rooted in the experience of antiblackness in the Americas, privileges a focus on enslavement and its aftermaths. The colonial experience and its ties to antiblackness remain under-researched, but are most likely to be found in the postcolonial work of Frantz Fanon, Achille Mbembe, Aimé Césaire and, more recently, Jemima Pierre. This book is written at the intersection of both iterations of Black Studies. As a consequence, while the concept of anti-blackness is central to this book, I focus on its colonial iterations. In doing so I bridge the divide between analyses of antiblackness on the western side of the Atlantic and those of colonial and racist violence on its eastern shores. The transatlantic, in my analysis, exceeds East–West mobilities, to include journeys from South to North and vice versa. British ships carried around one third of all those enslaved across the Atlantic; their routes linking Great Britain to the north to West Africa to the south, to the Americas in the west. Rather than focusing on the latter, *Antiblack-ness and Global Health* focuses in particular on antiblack mobilities linking the United Kingdom to Sierra Leone, both of which were important hubs during the trade in enslaved Africans. No one can undo the middle passage but, as Jemima Pierre (2013) has argued, bridging the (analytical) divide between experiences of racism and (anti)-Blackness on either side of the Atlantic contributes to calling out the workings of white supremacy on a global level.

The traditional remit of Black Studies, spanning the humanities and social sciences, means that the question of 'the human' has been closely attended to with regard to its social ontology and representations in liter-ature, anthropology, sociology and history. However, this remit has also precluded in-depth analyses of the perceived universality of the human in health and medical sciences. As with a Black Studies critique of con-ceptions of the human and the social in humanities and social sciences, Blackness has been excluded from medical and clinical conceptions of what it means to be human. Andrew Curran's (2011) work on Enlighten-ment anatomy and its role in justifying the exclusion of Blackness from white humanity speaks to the ways in which biomedicine and the dis-ciplines it builds on have deep entanglements with antiblackness. The modern justification for the continued exclusion of Blackness from med-ical practice is one of perceived colour-blindness: that all bodies are biologically the same and that therefore, the white, cis-heteronormative able-bodied male body can easily be used as stand-in for all other bodies, to the detriment of disabled, queer, women and Black, Indigenous and People of Colour (BIPOC) bodies. Such a conceptualisation excludes the fact that not all people share the same approach to and understanding of human biology, bodily health and illness. It also refuses to acknowl-edge that medical sciences, like social sciences, are relational, and that biomedicine has never treated all bodies equally. A contemporary example of how deeply foundational this exclusion is to modern practices of medicine is illustrated by Malone Mukwende et al.'s (2020) *Mind the Gap* handbook, the first clinical handbook focusing on how diseases present on dark skin. As Mukwende argued in an interview, medical textbooks circulate from Europe and North America to Africa, where medical students use the same books to study medicine (Jolie, 2021). Mukwende et al.'s handbook will be the first clinical handbook available to many African students which accurately depicts clinical symptoms on skin tones that represent those of their patients.

Antiblackness exceeds antiblack racism. It encompasses at once distinct eras/events that exemplify antiblack violence such as colonialism and the transatlantic slave trade as well as the antiblack racism that contributed to their realisation. It designates the structures, institutions and discourses, and the underlying attitudes, patterns and conditions that negate, or work to negate, Black life and humanity. As Costa Vargas and Jung (2021) write, antiblackness is tied to our conceptualisations of the human and the social and the latter's rejection of Blackness and Black people. They argue (2021, p. 7) that 'antiblackness [i]s an ontological condition of possibility of modern world sociality, whereas racism is an aspect of that sociality.' Antiblackness characterises antiblack weather, as defined by Sharpe (2016), and manifests itself in the hold; it is the wake. Antiblack racism takes place within it.

This book deals with antiblackness because the Ebola epidemic in Sierra Leone affected predominantly, and almost exclusively, Black people, in this case, people of African descent, and because antiblackness has shaped and been shaped by colonial British health interventions in Sierra Leone historically. Africans don't always identify as Black and, though central to colonialism, processes of racialisation and analyses thereof have long been the remit of diaspora studies rather than being seen as relevant to the sociology of the continent. Here I argue that the same processes of racialisation which shaped the emergence of modern Black subjects in the Americas, played out during the colonial and postcolonial era in sub-Saharan Africa. Antiblackness, this book argues, affects not only those who were enslaved, but depends on the conditions of enslaveability, and fungibility (Hartman, 1997), which affect Black/African life everywhere. In this book, when I write about Blackness I write about being African or of African descent. Perhaps, I could have called this book 'Anti-Africanness and Global Health', but intellectually Blackness continues to be a powerful currency. That too is a product of colonialism.

Antiblackness and Health

One may be misled into thinking that the question of Black humanity, central to the field of Black Studies, has long ago been settled for medicine and global health and thus does not need rehashing. European biomedicine, which global health relies on for its planning, analysis and evaluation, presents us with a universal *human* being; a model of the body and of health, structured around binary conceptions (and increasingly, gradations) of the normal and its deviations which is disproportionately based on the European male body. Skin colour, we are rightfully told, is not an indication of biological or clinical difference. Human medicine treats the human body regardless of its colour. But even in medicine there continues to be that niggling sense of doubt: are we all the same? The pseudoscientific attempts to link skin colour, and Black skin colour in particular, to racial difference, to establish hierarchies of humanity are deeply rooted in the development of Western medicine and continue on the fringes of mainstream science. Every so often they threaten to spill over (Saini, 2019). In the seventeenth and eighteenth centuries, European medicine, enabled by its colonial expansionism and industrial enslavement, began to consider race, not the environment, as the foundation for bodily and mental differences, including the propensity to ill health (Sowemimo, 2023). As the history of medicine shows, such views were not always relegated to the discipline's fringes. Sub-disciplines, such as craniology or phrenology, thrived in a world in which antiblackness had become institutionalised through colonialism and enslavement. Medical research, from the fifteenth to the twenty-first century could make use of Black bodies precisely because they were not seen as human, and could use them to scientifically demarcate their difference from white Europeans. Lundy Braun's (2014) detailed history of the spirometer, for instance, points to the tenacity and malleability of antiblackness in medicine to this day. Deirdre Cooper Owens (2017) offers a critical analysis of the role enslavement played in the making of American gynaecology. In the history of medicine and of global health, whose precursors colonial and tropical medicine availed themselves of Black and Brown research subjects to advance and propagate what we now know as biomedicine, even the gradual acceptance of Black bodies as human, did not spell their humanity. 'Today the idea that some biological element of race is to blame for poor health, rather than other social factors such as widespread racism and white supremacy, continues to be perpetuated' (Sowemimo, 2023, pp. 29–30).

European medicine, in its modern iteration has on the surface – as hard sciences often do – successfully disengaged from its murky, antiblack pasts, to make us forget that modern medicine is built on the non-consensual research and experimentation on Black bodies enabled by colonialism and enslavement. Medicine's antiblack past, when it is considered at all, is often seen as separate and unrelated to its modern practice. Modern medicine operates on the basis of the universal human body. The centrality of the human body and the universality of its clinical workings are, I would argue, one of the reasons why health and medicine only reluctantly engage with the broader historical, political and socio-economic dynamics that make this world. The problem that this book centres on is that, in global health and medicine, a Black body can be seen as human without Blackness being afforded the privilege of conceptual inclusion in humanity. This leads to delays in treatment, to a reluctance to administer pain medication and to different standards of health care. On a global scale it leads to vertical programming, unethical research on Black bodies, undignified media representation and insufficient or inadequate resources for health infrastructures.

This disconnect between a Black body as human and Black inhumanity, which I argue contributes to the refusal in health and medical sciences to engage with antiblackness, lies at the centre of this book. This disconnect becomes especially apparent because global health spans the divide between social and medical sciences; because it deals with bodies in public, rather than on an operating table. In global public health, medical and health-related sciences become tools that are deployed to intervene in political environments. This makes the contention that medicine and health are apolitical infinitely more difficult. It also directs us towards a deeper engagement with the relation between medicine and the contestation of Black (in)humanity – in other words, the entanglements between medicine and public health and antiblackness.

Hence, while this is a book about a global public health response and colonial antiblackness it is first and foremost a book that analyses the dismissal of colonial antiblackness in global health. Alongside research in archives, the book treats Sierra Leone and the physical environment in which the Ebola response took place as an archive of antiblackness, one which was largely ignored by health responders and logistical managers tasked with setting up the response. This marginalisation or, as João Costa Vargas (2018) calls it, *denial of antiblackness,* underlies global health to this date. Relatedly, the book is an invitation to read a global health event by questioning the colonial grammar with which we usually write global health stories. In doing so, it follows Kathryn Yusoff's (2018) critical approach to studying the Anthropocene. The book is not the product of a shift in global public health discernment of the impact racism has on health and medical practice, caused by the disproportionate mortality rates of people of African and Asian descent in Europe and the Americas during the ongoing Coronavirus pandemic. The research on which this book is based was carried out between late 2015 and early 2019. Rather, this book was born out of lived experience of medical racism, a long-standing interest in the interplay of antiblack racism, health and space, and an attempt to make sense of the intangible, fleeting and obscure hauntings of antiblackness in global health and otherwise. It started with two questions. First: *Why are Black people in formerly colonised countries more likely to be left to die in epidemic emergencies?*

This to me seemed like an important precursor to answering questions on medical racism in the African diaspora, which, since the beginning of the Covid-19 pandemic, have received more attention. In our long walk towards medical justice, these hauntings and this question will remain, even after the public's attention has turned away. *Antiblackness and Global Health* attests to the *longue durée* of antiblackness and its ability to shape Black and white life in the present. It attests to the many ways in which global health politics and interventions are shaped by and through colonial antiblackness. In my commitment to making sense of antiblackness in global health, the book offers new perspectives on present-day epidemic interventions and the management thereof that take the often violent colonial history of public health and medicine in West Africa into account. Doing so provides for a fuller, more honest analysis of disproportionate Black death and dying in humanitarian crises.

The second question which motivated this project was the following: *What if we knew the Ebola response and global health interventions more broadly, from a Black point of view; one that knows of abjection and slow death and ontological negation, one that knows antiblackness as lived reality?*

In this book I attempt such a way of knowing. Knowing Blackness and antiblackness are never merely intellectual endeavours and should not be approached as such. Knowing antiblackness in global health requires a break with European epistemology, with the illusion of distanced and objective, unfelt knowledge production. It requires a way of knowing global health, and the experience thereof that is empathic to the violent histories of (health) care in formerly colonised countries and to the depth of the entanglement between antiblackness and global health in the present while being acutely aware of the presence of joy and resistance and agency in relation to African health.

A Grammar of Refusal

I struggled with writing a beginning to this book. Beginnings are always the hardest parts to write. Finding the right words and tone, the right opener to this book was particularly difficult, possibly because it seemed, even to myself, like an impossible task. How to bring two fields so distinct into conversation with one another? Global health presents as technical and straightforward, medicine as universal and objective; Black Studies is differently universal. It is situated and emotive; embodied and radical. And yet, the disconnect between the two fields is an artificial one: (anti-) Blackness and modern conceptualisations and practices of medicine and health have always interacted and have always been interdependent. Moreover, this disconnect is one actively constructed by European knowledge production and epistemic coloniality. The fear I felt in sitting down to write this book, was largely related to the fear of committing what Walter Mignolo (2009) calls *epistemic disobedience*.

I commit several acts of epistemic disobedience in this book. The biggest of these consists in using Black Studies to analyse a global health event. In doing so I rupture the boundaries between hard and social sciences, between descriptions and experiences of a technical event and its broader programme effects, and the reality of the wake of colonialism and the transatlantic slave trade. In doing so the book follows Tiffany Lethabo King's (2019) writing in refusing 'to silo or treat intellectual traditions as bounded'. This book becomes an evaluation of a global health event through recourse to critical writings on antiblackness and colonialism. I ignore disciplinary boundaries to bring separate analytical and practical fields into conversation with one another. On the one side stands health as praxis, bounded by the belief in the universality of humanness, modelled on the experience of white European men. Black Studies, on the other hand, has long contested this idea. Indeed, some of its central fields of analysis are concerned with the fungibility of Black life and its exclusion from the category of *human*. Sylvia Wynter (2003), most prominently, has argued against the over-representation of European Man as a sign of the coloniality of power. By analysing a global health event through the prism of Black Studies I offer an analysis of the 2014–16 British-led international Ebola response from a Black perspective in order to undo the epistemic 'moves to innocence' which underlie European knowledge production (Tuck and Yang, 2012) and which, I contend, are particularly strong in global health and medicine. How have these moves to innocence protected global public health from a critical engagement with antiblackness? As the Decolonising Global Health movement has shown,[3] Black, Indigenous and other People of Colour perspectives are still marginal in dominant global health discourses and continue to be marginal in the design, conceptualisation and implementation of global health responses. As such, the book brings together two fields with radically opposed approaches in order to introduce the messy realities of antiblackness – seen and unseen, tangible and intangible, straightforward and haunted – into an analysis of global health, which survives through the measurement of metrics and hard facts, which continues to distance itself from social sciences and humanities. This then, is part theoretical exploration, part radically Black evaluation of an epidemic intervention.

The second act of epistemic disobedience consists in displacing Black Studies to work towards a theory of colonial antiblackness; to work towards an analysis of African experiences of antiblackness in relation to sub-Saharan Africa, rather than the Americas. In displacing Black Studies, this book engenders a conversation between two regions on terms of redress rather than violence. Black Studies is still firmly entrenched in the Americas, whereas much of global health is concerned with Africa. To make sense of, if not the merger then the rapprochement of these two fields requires an understanding of histories of racialisation and the making of Blackness between Africa and the Americas. As Jemima Pierre wrote: 'A modern, postcolonial space is invariably a racialised one; it is a space where racial and cultural logics continue to be constituted and reconstituted in the images, institutions and relationships of the structuring colonial moment' (2013, xii). This second act of disobedience, then, aims to establish an archive of colonial antiblackness that documents the violence of the past while also bearing witness to the complexities of the present. History, as Dionne Brand (2002) writes in *A Map to the Door of No Return*, rather than a void, is what we're born into, whether we like it or not. 'History', as Maya Angelou writes in her (2002) poem *On the Pulse of*

Morning, 'despite its wrenching pain cannot be unlived, but if faced with courage, need not be lived again'.

Sierra Leone, and West Africa more broadly, in the Western perception have long been viewed and understood through a lens tinged with medical racism. In 1836, F. Harrison Rankin, a member of the Royal Geographical Society (RGS, 1836, p. iix) published his book *The White Man's Grave: A Visit to Sierra Leone, in 1834* (Rankin, 1836), in which he described Sierra Leone as 'a colony little visited and little known, but, like all matters little known, the ground of much theory'. The role that Sierra Leone has played in shaping Western imaginations of West Africa and its inhabitants has always been linked to the political integration of Sierra Leone and West Africa more broadly into the global economy of the transatlantic. West Africa, especially, has also been closely linked to the history and establishment of tropical and colonial medicine, and political and academic institutions which continue to shape decision making in global health to this day. Antiblackness reaches from the past into the present and the future, and ensures a continuation of colonial power dynamics in global health. This book employs a grammar that forces an engagement with such history to tell new stories of an epidemic response.

Book Structure

This book's structure moves between the past and the present, between Sierra Leone, and specifically the Freetown Peninsula, the UK and the broader transatlantic. This non-linearity speaks to the complex and ever-shifting nature of antiblackness in our modern world, and to the ways in which a local West African event was shaped by European and global power structures. The chapters foreground various aspects of the entanglements between colonial antiblackness and global health politics, using the example of the British-led international EVD (Ebola virus disease) response in Sierra Leone. Chapter 1 materialises the colonial wake geographically on the Freetown Peninsula and points to the long-standing intersections between biomedical care and antiblack violence in and in relation to Sierra Leone. Chapter 2 focuses on the making of Blackness and antiblackness through the mobilities connecting Sierra Leone to the transatlantic and the UK, in particular in relation to historical and contemporary infectious disease controls. The chapter shows that the differential conceptualisation of mobilities linking Sierra Leone and the UK has long contributed to a reading of Sierra Leonean Blackness as risky, dependent and deviant on the one hand and entrepreneurial, independent and value-generating on the other. Chapter 3 casts a closer look at Ebola treatment centres and the spatial and temporal rhythms of infection prevention and control protocols. It shows that, in Sierra Leone, these rhythms reinforced the ambiguous and conditional inclusion of Black Sierra Leoneans into European conceptualisations of humanity and ordered patients into a spatial and racialised hierarchy. It also presents care for Black life as an antidote to that violence. Finally, chapter 4 interrogates knowledge production and expertise in global health in relation to the West African EVD epidemic and the research project that this book is based on. It shows that, as elsewhere, antiblackness was painfully obvious, and at times literally inescapable, in researching the international response to Sierra Leone's EVD epidemic, yet that it was largely sidelined in expert discussions and the management of the epidemic response, and that global structural inequalities reinforced the role of Europe as epistemic centre and whiteness as embodiment of expertise.

1

Place, Weather and Disease Control in (Post)Colonial Freetown

Introduction: Remains

On my second trip to Sierra Leone in March 2019 I am determined to visit the remains of Kerry Town Ebola treatment centre (ETC), which was financed by the British government and built by the British and Sierra Leonean armed forces. Kerry Town, of course, is more than a treatment centre: it's a village on the Freetown Peninsula. But for me and many others unfamiliar with pre-Ebola Sierra Leone, its first association is with the Ebola epidemic and the British and Sierra Leonean response. Kerry Town ETC has not been in use for several years now. In the newspaper I see photos of derelict buildings and debris. The treatment centre has entered a stage of ruination. 'How evocative', I think.

We drive from Freetown through Hastings and Waterloo. The scenery becomes increasingly rural, small villages follow one another. I have only known this place through photos and retellings, I want to see it for myself. But when we arrive there is nothing. Just earth and the beginning of new structures. The government has removed the ruins and is building a medical warehouse. I walk around the site, but there is very little to indicate that there once was a treatment centre here: A single surgical glove, a scrap of paper that may have been a laboratory or patient form. Otherwise just earth and rubble. The past as is often the case, has left no mark on this place. There is no memorial here, no plaque, nothing. Only new beginnings, and the village.

In Sierra Leone, and in West Africa more broadly, health and the built environment have long been shaped by white interventions, perspectives and voices. The transatlantic slave trade, colonialism and postcolonial development have left visible and invisible traces on the landscape, on attitudes, politics and societal make-up. Some of these traces are easily discernible, others take active work to unearth, but all shaped the development of both the Ebola epidemic and international response. In this chapter I engage in wake work. Wake work is 'a theory and praxis of the wake; a theory and praxis of Black being in diaspora' (Sharpe 2016, p. 19). Sierra Leone, of course, is not the diaspora. It is located in West Africa, on the upper Atlantic coast, wedged between Guinea on the one side and Liberia on the other. But through its forceful integration into transatlantic enslavement and European colonialism, Sierra Leone has generated a diaspora which continues to influence life and politics in Sierra Leone. Beginning in the eighteenth century, it has also itself been the recipient of Black diasporas who have been instrumental in shaping the country's modern statehood and continue to be influential in its politics. Sierra Leone, I suggest, is firmly in the wake in a way that is both visceral and complex, and that extends and complicates American analyses of Black diaspora. In Sierra Leone, European colonisation of Africa and the transatlantic slave trade come together to make the wake. In Sierra Leone's (post) colonial landscape, Blackness translates into native-ness and African-ness. Care for Black African life structures this book and its various historical representations in the history of Sierra Leone are themes in this chapter. So, at the outset a warning: let us be suspicious of care, of its uses, its framing and its manifestations in the wake. In Sierra Leone and with regard to Black life, everything that has been called by its name has not been care and often its framing has concealed violence.

In Sierra Leone today, the wake manifests as it has done for centuries: through British involvement framed as humanitarianism. Britain's role in intentionally 'underdeveloping' Sierra Leone, in raiding its people and resources and creating a colonial afterlife, which would justify continued British intervention, has been obscured by the language of humanitarian aid and development. Sierra Leone, which became independent from Great Britain in 1961, still bears the traces of having been a British colony. As Sierra Leone's biggest development partner, the UK played instrumental roles in ending Sierra Leone's 1991–2002 civil war (Kamara, 2018), but also in curbing the spread of the Ebola epidemic by sending healthcare workers and pledging £230 million to the Ebola response (PAC, 2015). As such, Great Britain is present both in Sierra Leonean political and economic life, but also in more subtle and permanent ways in architecture, in Freetown's urban form and in street, landmark and place names. The aftermath of enslavement and colonialism in Sierra Leone takes on political as well as spatial form. The colonial implications of the international response to the Ebola epidemic in which each former colonial power intervened in the country it had once colonised (Chaulia, 2014) fell on spatially fertile ground. In Freetown and surrounding areas, places were already marked by the antiblack violence of the slave trade and the British intervention which ended it. In street signs and place names the abolition of the slave trade and founding of the Sierra Leone Company are framed in philanthropic terms and are largely commemorated divorced from British involvement in the preceding slave trade. I suggest that it is the decidedly humanitarian and philanthropic framing of British colonial and imperial interventions in Sierra Leone that has led to its memorialisation and normalisation in street signs and place names. The environment in which care, and medical care especially, are provided, matter if we are to understand the relation of the epidemic and subsequent response to the antiblackness of the wake.

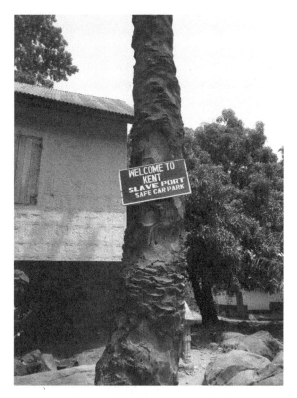

Figure 3   Sign indicating a safe parking spot in Kent, a village on the Freetown Peninsula: 'Welcome to Kent Slave Port. Safe Car Park'. (Photo by the author)

I took this photo (Figure 3) in Kent, a small fishing village about an hour from Freetown on my way to Banana Islands. Kent's history, as its name evokes, has long been entangled with the British presence in and influence on Sierra Leone. Like many other villages on the Freetown Peninsula, Kent was implicated in the slave trade in two ways: Portuguese slavers kept enslaved Africans here before transporting them on small boats to the nearby Banana Islands, in whose surrounding deep waters their slave ships could safely anchor. Later, after the abolition of the British slave trade, freed slaves founded the village of Kent and settled here (Leigh, 2016). Some material remains of the slave trade, such as the old St Edward's church, are still present, but today Kent is mostly known to foreigners for its sandy beaches and proximity to Banana Islands, both of which are attractive tourist destinations. The sign speaks to the normalisation of colonial and slave histories that have shaped the Freetown Peninsula. On the one hand it identifies Kent as a 'Slave Port', thereby attesting to the village's history in the transatlantic slave trade. On the other hand, it assures tourists that this is a safe parking spot, should they wish to leave their cars here before crossing over to Banana Islands or going to the beach. The fact that it is located right by the port, at the drop-off point for tourists wanting to cross to the Bananas, underlines this fact. It is where we park when we arrive. Here, antiblack legacies are leveraged and explicitly signalled to attract tourists interested in the history of the transatlantic slave trade in Sierra Leone. Simultaneously, the mention of Kent's historical reality as a slave port, next to the words 'Safe Car Park', trivialises the importance and long-lasting consequences of the transatlantic slave trade. Here, the safety of tourists' material possessions and the historical turning of Black life into possessions sit side by side, peacefully.

I approach the study of antiblackness by drawing on Sharpe's (2016) concepts of 'the wake' and 'the weather'. While Sharpe draws on the *Oxford English Dictionary* definition of weather and its meteorological elements (atmosphere, weather event, storm, etc.), she uses the term figuratively for poetic and aesthetic purposes. Sharpe uses Toni Morrison's (1987) *Beloved* to illustrate her conceptual use of weather. Morrison's protagonist Sethe is inspired by the story of Margaret Garner. Born into slavery, both the fictional Sethe and the real-life Margaret Garner kill their daughters to prevent them from being re-enslaved. In *Beloved*, Sethe and her surviving daughter Denver are haunted by the spirit of Sethe's dead child and by the past. Sharpe (2016, pp. 105–6) writes that:

[Sethe] wants to keep Denver from being overtaken by the past that is not past. Sethe wants to protect Denver from memory and from more than memory, from the experience, made material, of people and places that now circulate, like weather. [...] What Sethe remembers, rememories, and encounters in the now is the weather of being in the wake. [...] Slavery is imagined as a singular event even as it changed over time and even as its duration expands into supposed emancipation and beyond. But slavery was not singular; it was, rather, a singularity – a weather event or phenomenon likely to occur around a particular time, or date, or set of circumstances. Emancipation did not make Black life free; it continues to hold us in that singularity. The brutality was not singular; it was the singularity of antiblackness.

Sharpe describes slavery as a weather event. In this chapter I argue that antiblackness, in the case of Sierra Leone, circulates and manifests, not solely as a thing of the colonial and slave past, but because this past continues to hold Black Sierra Leoneans – and white international responders – in the present. The West African Ebola epidemic is one example of the ways in which Black life is held and shaped by antiblackness; it too is a weather event. The figurative use of weather and climate, two terms Sharpe largely uses interchangeably, contributes to the poetics of *In the Wake*. Like the weather, antiblackness is sometimes experienced intensely, sometimes barely noticed, and here I point to instances of both. Sharpe's conceptualisation helps to analyse present-day antiblackness, which, like meteorological weather, can be more or less conspicuous.

Echoing Sylvia Wynter's (2006, n.p.) statement that 'we live in an anti-Black world' and seeking to confront the shifting tangibility of this antiblack world, Sharpe innovates with her conceptual reading of weather. She writes: 'In my text, the weather is the totality of our environments; the weather is the total climate; and that climate is antiblack' (2016, p. 104). For Sharpe, weather and climate are conceptual devices for thinking and writing about how antiblackness manifests in the wake. Focusing on Freetown and the Freetown Peninsula, this chapter explores the more or less conspicuous environments and climates in which the Sierra Leonean Ebola epidemic and response took place. I foreground remains of Sierra Leone's colonial and antiblack past and show how these created a spatial, epistemic, atmospheric and structural environment of antiblackness, reminiscent of Sharpe's antiblack wake and weather. Throughout the book I often refer to/describe things as 'colonial and antiblack'. In my text

I understand colonialism in Africa to be a manifestation of antiblackness. Consequently, I do not see the two as separate, but as a specific and general attribute of the phenomena I describe and analyse.

Colonial Aftermaths

Care and Colonial Remains

Few of us study the weather in detail. It just is. Only those directly affected by its effects, pay close attention to how it structures our lives, enables and curtails possibilities. Uncovering histories of Black liberation and of the antiblack structures in which they occur works along similar lines. It is entirely possible to move through downtown Freetown and only briefly notice the many reminders of the city's historical encounters with British expansionism, even if one is attuned to the structuring power of coloniality and antiblackness. Neighbourhoods, streets and waterways in Freetown bear names that recall British abolitionists, colonial officials and early settlers. When I first get to Freetown, every encounter with these jolts through me and fills me with excitement (see: the past is right *here*). I become less excited the longer I stay. With time the past becomes a normality, a location rather than a temporal marker, although sites remain, of course, both. Havelock Street, Wilberforce Street, Wilkinson Street, Macaulay Street, to name just a few, bear the names of British colonial governors, abolitionists and officials. Wilberforce Street (Figure 4) and the Wilberforce neighbourhood are named after William Wilberforce, the British abolitionist and one of the co-founders of the Sierra Leone Company. Wilkinson Road, one of the main roads in Freetown's West End in turn recalls the name of Moses Wilkinson, a former enslaved man and Black Nova Scotian who arrived in Sierra Leone in 1792 (Clifford, 2006). (I spend long mornings and afternoons on Wilkinson Road, sometimes zooming past, sometimes stuck in traffic on the way from Aberdeen, where I live temporarily, to the city centre.) Macaulay Street, too, is named after colonial officials: second cousins Zachary and Kenneth Macaulay both served, as Governor and Acting-Governor of the colony respectively, the first between 1794 and 1795 and 1796 and 1799, the second in 1826. A stream near the old boundary of Granville Town, one of the first settlements established by the formerly enslaved and free Blacks on the coast of Sierra Leone is called Granville Brook, after Granville Sharpe, perhaps the most ardent proponent of what he called the 'Province of Freedom' (Wilson, 1976). Today, one of Freetown's official waste disposal sites is named Granville Brook Dumpsite, after the brook (Sankoh et al., 2013). This stream (and the dumpsite) I only ever see on the map, my Freetown life revolves around the city centre and Freetown's West End.

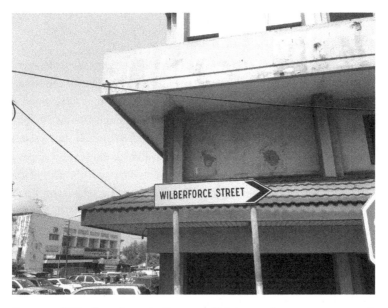

Figure 4   Wilberforce Street in Freetown. This is one of many streets named after British abolitionists or colonial officers. (Photo by the author)

One of the possible reasons for why these colonial remains endure, largely uncontested in Freetown's cityscape, is the historical framing of British colonialism. The latter was characterised by a framing of humanitarianism and benevolence, even more pronounced than in other African colonies (Fyfe, 1962; Frenkel and Western, 1988). Freetown was established as a settlement in 1792 on an initiative of the Sierra Leone Company, created by British abolitionists such as William Wilberforce and Granville Sharpe (Ingham and Clarkson, 1894). After the American War of Independence in 1783, Free Black Nova Scotians, Black loyalists, Jamaican Maroons and poor urban Black people from London and other cities across the British empire were settled in the new territory. An early company report from 1791 described the beginnings of the enterprise as follows:

About five years since, the streets of London swarming with a number of Blacks in the most distressed situation, who had no prospect of subsisting in this country but by depredations on the public, or by common charity, the humanity of some respectable Gentlemen was excited towards these unhappy objects. They were accordingly collected to the number of above 400, and, together with 60 Whites [...] they were sent out at the charge of government to Sierra Leone. (Sierra Leone Company, 1791, p. 3)

Following this first settlement, the Sierra Leone Company took it upon itself to gather funds to relocate more destitute Black people and to support the beginnings of their livelihoods in Sierra Leone. This brand of colonialism has been described as 'humanitarian imperialism' (Frenkel and Western, 1988; also Fyfe, 1962). In a later 'Report from the Committee on the Petition of the Court of Directors of the Sierra Leone Company' from 1802 (TNA [The National Archives] – WO1/352) the aim of the establishment of the Sierra Leone Company and the subsequent establishment of the settlement of Freetown are described thus: 'The general object of the founders of [the Company] was the introduction of civilisation into Africa.'

The history of Freetown's founding and its naming speak to differences in reading the past. According to British officials, the name Freetown was chosen by the Sierra Leone Company. Drawing on the diary of John Clarkson, Freetown's first governor, Ernest Graham Ingham (Ingham and Clarkson, 1894, p. 10), who served as Bishop of Sierra Leone at the end of the nineteenth century (Sibthorpe, 1970) described the founding and naming of Freetown thus: 'The land was cleared in a few weeks, and the town was named Freetown, in consequence of an instruction to that effect sent out from home.' 'Home' in this case refers to England, from which both Governor Clarkson and Reverend Ingham came.

The story of Freetown's creation is told differently in the city itself. A mural at the government-commissioned Sierra Leone Peace and Cultural Monument celebrates Thomas Peters, an enslaved man born in the North American colonies, who joined the British fight against American Independence and was freed and resettled in Sierra Leone, as the 'True Founder of Freetown'. Unsurprisingly, the story of Freetown's founding as told by the Sierra Leonean government differs from the nineteenth-century colonial governors' account. This discrepancy in Freetown's founding story, between the version recorded at The National Archives in Kew and the one etched into stone in Freetown's Peace and Cultural Monument, is indicative of the multiple histories and interpretations that coexist in the wake; histories that layer and obscure Black agency and exploitation.

Regardless of who Freetown's true founder was (both histories leave out indigenous Temne people living on the Freetown Peninsula), Freetown became, in the late eighteenth century, the British repatriation destination for Black people freed from enslavement. As such, Freetown was the first settlement of freed slaves from the Americas and the Caribbean established on the African continent (Olusoga, 2016). This is reflected in the toponymy of the colony and its capital.

Racial and Sanitary Segregation

Spaces are a representation of how we remember the past. At times they are a reflection of the passage of time: of how we have moved on and glorified the past, or sanitised it, or built on top of and around it or let it slip into oblivion – it's there, but we're too busy with the here and now to dwell on it. In Freetown, spatial remains exemplify the wake in correlation with contemporary disease management. I see these material remains as 'ruins' or 'debris' (Stoler, 2013, 2016). Rather than actual states of physical disrepair, these terms suggest colonial and imperial durabilities present in the physical remains and capable of shaping contemporary Black life. Stoler (2013, p. 12) describes her work on ruins and ruination as follows: 'Here we envision colonial histories of the present that grapple with the psychological weight of remnants, the generative power of metaphor, and the materiality of debris to rethink the scope of damage and how people live with it.'

As the excerpt from the 1913 map of Freetown (Figure 5) shows, street names are not the only feature through which the colonial past is visible in Freetown today. Colonial urban design both translated and masked the urban realisation of racial and class segregation (Legg, 2007). In Freetown's urban form, especially the colonial-style architecture (Figure 6) scattered across the city (Stone, 2012; Akam, 2012) and its grid system (visible in Figure 5), are reminders of the colonial origins of the city and the racial segregation that was inherent to its spatial logic. The grid system according to which Freetown's city centre is organised is a typical example of British colonial town layout, as it afforded easy military access and administrative governability (Brockett, 1998). The centrality of military barracks (Figure 5) and the spatial and physical difference between settler and native towns (Fanon, 1965) is also observable in Freetown. Colonial

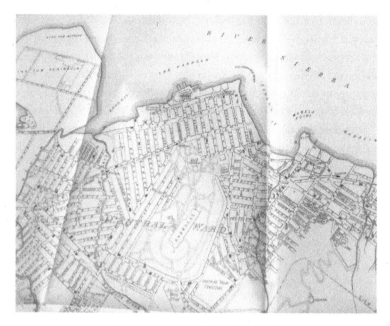

Figure 5   Excerpt of Freetown map 1913. The Colonial Hospital is situated in the top centre, just off Oxford Street. (TNA – CO 270/45)

houses were built in enclaves, often located on hills and away from downtown Freetown. Two of these enclaves, Wilberforce and Hill Station, have been highlighted in Figure 6. The location of the settler towns is traceable through prevailing colonial-style architecture in Freetown. A high number of colonial homes are still situated in the Wilberforce and Hill Station neighbourhoods (Stone, 2012; Akam, 2012; Doherty, 2015). These remains, like Stoler's (2013) ruins, give the colonial past a material present in relation – and in proximity – to which life in Freetown plays out. In Freetown, a history of healthcare is intricately interwoven with these colonial ruins.

Hill Station in Freetown, named and modelled after the Indian model of sanitary segregation (Lewis, 1954; Cole, 2014), was built for colonial officers and their wives in what was considered to be a cooler, healthier climate than downtown Freetown in 1902 (Frenkel and Western, 1988). (The caption below the 1871 photo of a Hill Station House – Figure 6 – mentions the temperature varying between 68° and 77° Fahrenheit, that is, 20–25° Celsius, which was cooler than downtown Freetown. The temperatures in Hill Station are still on average lower than in the city centre.)

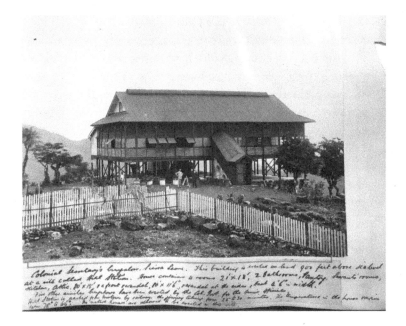

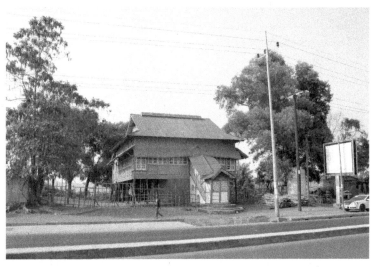

Figure 6   Example of British colonial architecture in Hill Station, Freetown in 1871 and 2019. The bottom line of the description reads 'No native houses are allowed to be erected in this site.' (Top photo, TNA – CO1069/88; bottom photo by the author)

Rather than following Ronald Ross's advice to invest in a city-wide drainage system (this would reduce the amount of stagnant puddles used by *Anopheles* mosquitoes as breeding grounds), which the colonial government deemed too costly, Governor King-Harman opted for urban segregation (Fyfe, 1962). The relocation of government staff entangled racial segregation with sanitary segregation and introduced both into the urban landscape. In Roy Lewis's book *Sierra Leone: A Modern Portrait* (1954), he described this entanglement: 'So Hill Station was built, and the officials began to move up; and in 1902 the creole doctors (who stayed down, with their patients) were relegated to inferior positions in the new West African Medical Service' (Lewis, 1954, p. 167). Christopher Fyfe (1962, p. 611) described the changes to Freetown's urbanism thus:

> While all were neighbours in Freetown, while the Chief Justice lived in a flat over an undertaker's warehouse, the Colonial Secretary in the battered old Secretariat, neighbourhood interests bound Europeans and Africans. They broke when one racial group was isolated in the hills with wire fences and threatening notices to keep out the other. Thus the Indian model of racially stratified society was introduced into Sierra Leone, not shamefacedly as required by prejudice, but openly as dictated by medical science.

Hill Station's origin – it retains its name to this day – is one of racial segregation and medical racism. To protect colonial officers from becoming infected with malaria, they were encouraged to sleep away from native populations who were deemed to be harbouring disease. 'Native' houses and people were not considered to be sanitary, but rather were seen to be host to mosquitoes and other organisms capable of transmitting tropical diseases to colonising populations (Frenkel and Western, 1988) thereby confirming Fanon's (1965, pp. 38) declaration that 'the native town [...] is a place of ill fame'. At the start, no native houses were allowed to be erected in Hill Station and Black servants were only allowed to remain on Hill Station for short periods of time (Fyfe, 1962; Spitzer, 1968).

In the annual medical reports, in which data on the health of the colony was collected and which were then sent to London, a special section was dedicated to Hill Station. In a 1910 report by the medical department in Sierra Leone the general health of the site is discussed as follows:

The health conditions of Hill Station have during 1910 continued to be quite satisfactory. [...] The total number of cases on the sick list was 18. Of these 6 were due to climatic causes: -

Malarial Fever	5
Yellow Fever (suspected)	1

In three of the cases of Malaria Fever, infection was contracted during visits to out-stations in the Protectorate. Two of the cases occurred in the Military residents who worked in Freetown daily. The suspected case of Yellow Fever occurred in a newly arrived official who frequently had to remain in his office overtime, owing to extra work, and was not, in consequence, able to leave Freetown until late in the afternoon. [...] The only non-official residences up to the present are the General's, Cable Company's and the Wesleyan Mission's, none of the Mercantile firms of Freetown having so far taken the advantage of the undoubted claims of Hill Station as a healthier place of residence for Europeans as compared with the climatic and present sanitary conditions prevailing in the town. (TNA – CO 270/45, p. 16)

In the report, Freetown, meaning downtown Freetown, is constructed as a (Black) 'native' place of disease, whereas Hill Station is a (white) 'European' place of health. Neither the name Hill Station nor the medical report indicate the racial component of the urban and sanitary management of Freetown and the role that Hill Station played in both. Rather, the report painstakingly lists the places of infection with malaria and yellow fever as having occurred in places other than Hill Station: in downtown Freetown, the protectorate and among those who worked in Freetown daily, thereby reinforcing the link between Blackness, place and disease. The imaginaries underlying Freetown's urban layout remain largely unchanged. Although no longer an exclusively white neighbourhood, Hill Station is still a highly coveted living space. The president's residence is located here, as are a number of embassies. When the British-led IMATT (the International Military Advisory and Training Team) moved to Freetown to advise the Republic of Sierra Leone Armed Forces at the end of the civil war in 2001, they moved to Hill Station (Gberie, 2017). This further consolidated Hill Station's status as a secure living space for elite Sierra Leoneans (Akam, 2012; Gberie, 2017), an impression further cemented when the Americans built a $40 million embassy on the site (Gberie, 2017). The exclusive status conferred upon Hill Station by British colonial officers who settled here for health reasons and turned it into a white-only area, lives on in the wake of colonialism: in preserved colonial houses, but also in British and American military presence and elevated real estate prices.

Freetown's urban form displays an uneasy and complex relationship with colonialism, which lays the groundwork for an uneven urban landscape, and in which life occurs amid colonial ruins. Although not technically in ruins (see Stoler, 2013), Hill Station exemplifies the hold the colonial past has on the present in that it continuously embodies the exclusivity that colonial officers intended for it. Its de facto exclusion no longer operates on the basis of racial and ethnic characteristics, but today takes on a more classed and capitalist character.

Biomedicine and Antiblackness

In order to understand how the Ebola response played out in the colonial wake, we need to think antiblackness as 'the ground on which we stand' (Sharpe, 2016, p. 7). One corner of Freetown illustrates the historical relationship between spatial remains, antiblackness, disease management and care: Connaught Hospital, Freetown's main adult referral hospital (KSLP, 2019). The hospital is named after the Duke of Connaught, who visited Freetown shortly before the hospital was completed at the beginning of the twentieth century. The antiblackness that has long been entangled with care in this site, has been physically erased, enabling a reading of Sierra Leonean history that valorises British humanitarianism and care. Connaught Hospital, as this section shows, quite literally stands on grounds that have long been shaped by antiblackness. Writing about medical care in (post)colonial Africa, necessitates caring about the antiblack violence that has historically shaped this corner of Freetown in particular. For centuries colonialism and the resettlement of the enslaved in and around Freetown have been framed as philanthropic gestures of care, obscuring how antiblackness took place here.

The site on which Connaught Hospital is located, on the northern edge of Freetown, has long been a place in which care and violence have coincided. In the period from 1690 to 1800 between 440,000 and 660,000 enslaved Africans were shipped to the Americas from the coast of Sierra Leone (Rodney, 1980, pp. 250–1; Shaw, 2002, p. 29). The majority of slave ships sailed under a British flag (Trans-Atlantic Slave Trade Database, 2019). With the abolition of the British slave trade in 1807, the British Navy patrolled the coast of West Africa, captured slave ships, and brought the enslaved to King's Yard, an enclosed space on the site that Connaught Hospital now occupies and which used to be the location of the Colonial Hospital (Fyfe, 1962; TNA – CO 270/45). In King's Yard, the enslaved were registered and medically examined by British Navy doctors and officers. For a short while and if necessary, they were cared for in the adjoining Royal Hospital and Asylum (Olusoga, 2016, pp. 309–10), before the latter was moved to Regent, and at times isolated, to protect the health of the colony, before being resettled in and around Freetown.[1] Thus for many freed slaves, Western biomedicine and confinement marked the transition from enslavement to resettlement and the promise of liberation. Ironically, the most detailed written account of King's Yard and life therein at the apogee of the nineteenth-century British Courts of Mixed Commissions is delivered to us by F. Harrison Rankin, the author of *The White Man's Grave: A Visit to Sierra Leone* (1836). Rankin, who according to Fyfe (1962) was a clerk in the Courts of Mixed Commission, but who presented himself as an independent traveller, was opposed to the trade in enslaved Africans and his book was meant to convey a more accurate and generous depiction of Sierra Leone hitherto often referred to by Europeans as 'the white man's grave' but described by Rankin (1836, p. 3) as 'the asylum of the unfortunate and the adopted land of civilisation'. Despite his opposition to the slave trade and to the form the liberation of enslaved Africans took in Sierra Leone, Rankin's attitudes towards Black Africans were typically racist and paternalistic and, although he described Black criticisms of Britain's colonial politics in his book, he remained a firm believer in the superiority of British civilisation and the civilising and humanitarian function of British colonialism in Sierra Leone.

Rankin was an eyewitness to both the bureaucratic and actual processes of liberation. Although Great Britain passed legislation to end the British slave trade in 1807, their treaties with other slave-trading nations were conditional. Some extended the legality of trading in enslaved Africans until a point in the future (1826 for Brazilian ships, 1829 for Dutch), for others the 'inhuman trade' was prohibited only between specific latitudes (Rankin, 1836, p. 95). Ships caught by the British Navy outside those latitudes had to be released and could continue their journey without hindrance, condemning enslaved Africans onboard to a future of violence and death. Both conditions, often obscured in official British accounts of the abolition of transatlantic enslavement, speak to the geographical and temporal restrictions placed on African humanity and the ways in which the 1807 Slave Trade Act legalised these restrictions.

Detained ships would be towed into Freetown Harbour and Africans on board would eventually be brought to a space called the King's Yard. Rankin, as a clerk of the Courts of Mixed Commission, spent considerable amounts of time in King's Yard and described the processes of liberation in his book (1836, pp. 106–30):

> On condemnation [of the ship], the slaves are adopted as British free subjects, are landed, and conveyed, in the first instance, to the King's Yard, a large species of prison, consisting of a central house, within a square yard, surrounded by open sheds; the whole encompassed by high walls, and secured by well-guarded gates. [...] The captives remain in the King's Yard, in rather equivocal freedom, until formally disposed of: each, when landed, is furnished with a slight, partial covering. The men, boys, and girls receive about a yard and a quarter of coarse white cotton wrapper; the women put on a check garb, simply sewed at the sides, with holes for the arms, and extending from the neck to the knees. After a few days, the whole are freed, to make room for successors. In this wise freedom visits the captives. The men are inspected by a sergeant and officer when conscripts are wanted. The most muscular are drafted at once into the King's service; and are marched in a string, nolentes volentes, under strong barracks, to learn regimental discipline.

Rankin's descriptions emphasise the antiblackness that suffused the moment of liberation itself. In order to deal with the legal aspects of emancipation, handled by the Courts of Mixed Commission, the enslaved had to await their fate in a prison and were subsequently liberated in batches. The men were commonly directly drafted into the British military, thus marking the beginning of another form of servitude. Fanon (1988 [1952]), in the context of independence struggles across Africa, offered a pertinent critique of Black liberation, which seems particularly relevant to the descriptions of King's Yard offered by Rankin: 'Historically, the Black Man steeped in the inessentiality of servitude was set free by his master. [...] The upheaval reached the Black Man from without. The black man was acted upon.' In the context of King's Yard, freedom was bestowed upon enslaved Africans through British legal processes and treaties, once again undermining African pre-enslavement and pre-colonial sovereignty and agency. Rankin next went on to describe the *liberation* of women and children:

The women are submitted for choice to such negroes as express desire for conjugal happiness; and are carried off to joy by liege lords, who assume their unmasked consent, under the sanction of the Governor. Short is the courtship; for the languages of the pair are generally unintelligible to each other. Few are the throbs of anxiety, and light the labours of wooing, where the ladies' will is not consulted. In the negro vocabulary of love 'wife' signifies servant and labourer, tiller of the ground, grinder of corn, water-bearer. The captive women are eagerly pounced upon as wives.

The children under fourteen now remain to be emancipated from the horrors of slavery. Any resident in the colony, of any colour, may enter the King's Yard, select a girl or a boy, and thereupon tie a string or piece of tape round the neck as a mark of appropriation. He then pays ten shillings; and the passive child becomes his property, under the name of apprentice, for three years.

Rankin's account clearly shows how conceptualisations of Black/African people as outside of humanity pervaded not only enslavement but also the processes of abolition. These processes took spatial form in the King's Yard and are contributing factors to the history not only of Sierra Leone, but also of the site that Connaught Hospital is situated on. His next observations are particularly relevant with regard to health and healthcare in Sierra Leone and King's Yard/Connaught Hospital as a site in which antiblackness and biomedicine coincide:

To the King's Yard I paid frequent visits, and found an interest awakened in behalf of the people. The young children soon recovered from their sufferings, and their elastic spirits seemed little injured. The men next rallied; but several died in the shed devoted to the most sickly, chiefly from dysentery: they were wrapped in a coarse grass mat, carried away, and buried without ceremony. Of the women many were despatched to the hospital at Kissy, victims to raging fever; others had become insane. I was informed that insanity is the frequent fate of the women captives, and that it chiefly comes upon such as at first exhibit most intellectual development, and greatest liveness of disposition.

Again, Rankin's observations give us an inkling of life in King's Yard shortly after its establishment. The site that now hosts a hospital, used to be a prison for the assessment and later dispersal of Africans *rescued* from enslavement by those who had previously enslaved them. The conditions and processes of African/Black inclusion into the realm of who counts and who does not count as human, remain with the British. Healthcare seems to have been a feature of this site since its inception and the ways in which the coincidence of healthcare and antiblackness shaped the history and present of this site interests me to this day. Today, the only physical remains of King's Yard is one of two original gates, which stands on the grounds of Connaught Hospital (Figure 8). Erected in 1817 by Governor McCarthy, the gate marked the boundary to King's Yard. The gate still opens up into a yard, albeit a small one, leading to an eye clinic and the back door of the hospital's department of internal medicine. On some days, parts of the yard are used for Muslim prayers. Its uses have changed. An original inscription at the top of the gate (see Figure 7) references the Royal Hospital and Asylum that was constructed to provide care to 'Africans rescued from slavery by British valour and philanthropy' and thereby attests to the history of British care in this site.[2] King's Yard forms a spatial and political marker of the transition from enslavement to resettlement in Sierra Leone. Once landed in King's Yard, the African names of the 'recaptives' were usually discarded, marking a further stripping of their identities, and many adopted the names of missionaries or masters later on (Fyfe, 1962). Today the gate is just a gate, its use functional and not necessarily commemorative for the everyday workings of Connaught Hospital. However, resettlement did not mean freedom. It often entailed further unpaid labour for up to 14 years under the so called 'apprenticeship system' (Fyfe, 1961; Olusoga, 2016, p. 314), a practice that many Africans criticised (Rankin, 1836). Rankin described an exchange with a Susu man in his book, one of the few Black voices we hear from in his account:

Knowing him to be much attached to the English, I put the question whether he would refuse to fight if the Timmanees were to make another attack upon the town. 'Yes, he would fight for the white men' he said ; 'but would not be a slave.' I asked him what he meant by slave; the word had not been mentioned. 'Soldiers,' he answered, 'are slaves; loaded with heavy arms and dress, shut up in the barracks as if it were the goal, forced to march and labour against their will when the white men pleased;' and, finally to clinch his argument he exclaimed, 'they make soldiers of Captives;' that is, of the Liberated slaves. Nothing could modify his opinion and the opinion of the Soosoo was the prevalent one.

In the site, now occupied by Connaught Hospital, antiblackness both preceded and followed biomedical care.

King's Yard functioned as a prison and hospital for Africans transitioning from enslavement to freedom until 1844, shortly after which the Liberated African Hospital became the Colonial Hospital (Fyfe, 1962). The Royal Hospital and Asylum/Colonial Hospital was torn down in the

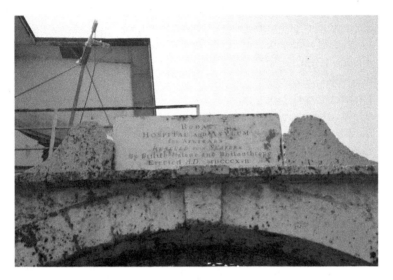

Figure 7   Original plaque on top of King's Yard Gate. (Photo by the author)

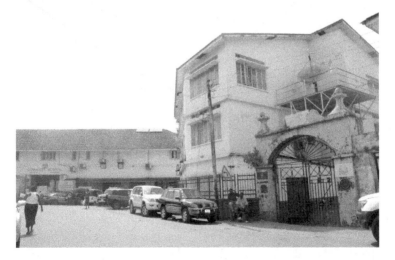

Figure 8   Connaught Hospital and King's Yard Gate. (Photo by the author)

early twentieth century. A 1913 Annual Medical Report on Sierra Leone describes the plans for its demolition and for the subsequent construction of Connaught Hospital, which was built on the site in the 1920s, after part of the Colonial Hospital burnt down (TNA – CO270/45, p. 97; TNA – CO1071/323, p. 21) and was named for the Duke of Connaught who visited Sierra Leone in 1910 (TNA – CO1069/88/241).[3] Today the only physical remains of the histories of enslavement and liberation at this site are reminders of British care: Connaught Hospital itself and the gate to King's Yard, whose plaque recalls 'British valour and philanthropy'. What remains (Connaught Hospital, King's Yard Gate) after colonial domination offers insights into the strategic tenacity of colonialism's afterlife. I extend Stoler's (2013) argument by suggesting that these remains also show the conscious erasure of histories of antiblackness. The reminder of 'British Valour and Philanthropy' atop King's Yard Gate on the grounds of Connaught Hospital obscures the antiblackness that made Britain a major benefactor and proponent of the transatlantic slave trade in the first place. It also erases the antiblack sentiment that led to the stipulation in the 1807 Act for the Abolition of the Slave Trade, giving to:

His Majesty, His Heirs and Successors, and such Officers, Civil or Military, as shall, by any general or special Order of the King in Council, be from Time to Time appointed and empowered to receive, protect, and provide for such Natives of Africa as shall be so condemned [to slavery], [the power] either to enter and enlist the same, or any of them, into His Majesty's Land or Sea Service, as Soldiers, Seamen, or Marines, or to bind the same, or any of them, whether of full Age or not, as Apprentices, for any Term not exceeding Fourteen Years.[4]

Antiblackness structured the Act for the Abolition of the Slave Trade, in that it ensured the possibility for further Black servitude in Africa. This is reminiscent of what Mbembe (2001, p. 13) has termed European 'doubt of the very possibility of [African] self-government'. As during the colonial period, whose onset, in Sierra Leone, neatly coincided with the abolition of the slave trade, Africans, after leaving King's Yard Gate, were not free, but had to serve as apprentices to Black and white settlers (Fyfe, 1962). These histories of antiblackness are invisible in the physical remains of Connaught Hospital and King's Yard Gate. Making sense of these geographies of the wake, in which what remains and what is obscured extends colonial logics of Black dependency and British care, requires a consciousness of the versatile continuity of antiblackness today, and an acceptance that we live and care in the wake of colonialism and antiblackness. Although not visible in the physical remains of King's Yard, antiblackness continued to structure medical care in Sierra Leone. In the years following the abolition of the slave trade and the colonisation of Sierra Leone, care continued to be associated with this site in the form of the Colonial and then the Connaught Hospital. Healthcare, or rather care for the health of Europeans, was a crucial component of colonial governance in Sierra Leone. With the increasing propagation of social Darwinism, Freetown's social life, which throughout the first half of the nineteenth century had been relatively well integrated, at least within various social classes, became increasingly segregated. This development was further amplified by Ross's advances in malaria research and his findings, among those of other researchers, that the *Anopheles* mosquito, rather than diseased climates transmitted malaria. Given the presumed endemicity of malaria in the region and relative immunity from the disease that long-term (i.e. Black African) residents possessed, spatial segregation on sanitary terms was proposed and implemented at the beginning of the twentieth century and culminated in the establishment of Hill Station (Spitzer, 1968). Within the Colonial Hospital, the sanitary segregation that characterised Freetown's racialised residential organisation took hold as well. In 1910 Freetown experienced a yellow fever epidemic. A 1910 annual report by the colonial medical department details the isolation arrangements that were made to prepare the Colonial Hospital for infectious disease control:

Owing to the outbreak of Yellow Fever in the town during the month of May, it was found necessary to make arrangements for the isolation of patients suffering from, or suspected of suffering from this disease.

For this purpose the Matron's Cottage in the [Colonial] Hospital enclosure was divided into two rooms containing one bed each and was set apart for Europeans [...]. For the purpose of isolating natives at the Hospital, eleven beds on the male side and five beds on the female side were provided with mosquito netting. (TNA – CO 270/45, p. 19)

Thus, a century before the onset of the Ebola epidemic, biomedical care in Sierra Leone was characterised by racial segregation. Standards of care varied between those provisions taken to protect Europeans against yellow fever and those put in place for the Black 'native' population. As with the residential segregation at Hill Station, medical racism led to the establishment of a parallel yet unequal system of disease management. During the 1910 yellow fever epidemic, the mortality rate in the Sierra Leonean part of the hospital was higher than in the refurbished matron's cottage reserved for Europeans. Of 14 European patients isolated at the Colonial Hospital, 9 'recovered and returned to work. Four recovered and were invalided. One died (Yellow Fever)' (TNA – CO270/45, p. 19). On the 'native' ward, on the other hand 'four cases admitted into these beds were diagnosed as Yellow Fever, three of them died [...]' (TNA – CO270/45, p. 19). Although anecdotal, these accounts speak to differential mortality rates that would be reproduced during the Ebola epidemic.

In 2014, as in 1910, Sierra Leoneans were cared for separately from European patients.[5] Anton, who worked for a British NGO during the Ebola response, commented on the impossibility of caring for Sierra Leonean health care workers infected with the virus in Kerry Town Ebola treatment centre: 'What would have been reassuring would have been that local health care workers could be treated in Kerry Town. And in the end, they never confirmed [that this would take place], they just did it on the side.'[6]

Anton was angry about this. Although his remark 'they just did it on the side' indicates that local–international, or Black/white, segregation was not strictly observed at Kerry Town, he was acutely aware of the anti-black tensions that permeate contemporary global health management and which translated into an uncertain access to care for Sierra Leonean healthcare workers. Dina, an epidemiologist who volunteered at Kerry Town also pointed to the racial segregation she observed in care arrangements during the Ebola epidemic. According to her account, one section of the treatment centre, was reserved for (predominantly white) expat healthcare workers. Commenting on the exclusivity of this part of the ETC she said (sarcastically): 'Now it's called health worker treatment [centre] but it used to be white worker treatment.' Dina acknowledged the underlying racial segregation in treatment facilities.

Here, as in other places, I found a discrepancy between what was done in practice, or what I was told, and what existed in the official record. It is in these gaps, that antiblackness manifests most commonly and into whose uncertainties it is relegated, when looking for proof. Racism and antiblackness were not officially put forward as reasons to dedicate one section of Kerry Town ETC to the care of (international) health care workers. Rather, in a letter to NHS (National Health Service) staff sent in September 2014, Dame Sally Davies, then chief medical officer of the UK and Professor Sir Bruce Keogh, then medical director of NHS England, wrote that:

> The treatment centre will comprise of a 12 bed unit for healthcare workers, *including any local or international medical volunteers*. It will provide high quality specialist care to ensure essential health workers can continue to respond to the disease as safely and efficiently as possible. A co-located 50 bed unit will be built for treating additional patients with the disease. This centre will be staffed by international health workers and staff from Sierra Leone, and will provide treatment to both adult and paediatric victims of the disease. (Davies et al., 2014; emphasis added)

On paper then, it seems as if instructions for the dedicated 12-bed treatment centre would have included 'local volunteers' but this seems to have been contested, confused or resisted in practice on the ground. In the historical context of British medical and sanitary segregation on racial grounds in Sierra Leone, these present-day confusions, hesitations and contested practices evoke the antiblackness of the past. At the same time, as the example of Connaught Hospital has shown, places of biomedical care have spatially coincided with antiblackness in Sierra Leone. I further explore this spatial coincidence towards the end of this chapter. In the wake, the antiblackness that permeated (medical) care in Sierra Leone, in terms of racial segregation and forced labour, has left no physical mark and takes work to unearth, yet the past resurfaces in uncomfortable and problematic ways.

In Freetown and the Freetown Peninsula, colonial remains continue to shape the city's urban form and contribute to making the wake a spatial reality through the city's urban design, in street and place names. The colonial rationale which influenced the street layout (Brockett, 1998), and the division between settler and native towns (Fanon, 1965), are still visible in Freetown's urban organisation yet the racial segregationist rationale that characterised colonial Freetown often remains obscured. The colonial past is normalised in street names and location markers that obscure the often violent and antiblack nature of the colonial enterprise in Sierra Leone behind discourses of care and humanitarianism. Like Sharpe's weather (2016), the antiblackness that characterises the wake is omnipresent in Freetown's urban form and the site of Connaught Hospital, yet also inconspicuous.

Discourses asserting Sierra Leone's founding as the first free Black settlement and as a place of Black liberation obscure the violence of the transatlantic slave trade in which British interests played a crucial role. As exemplified in the physical remains of King's Yard Gate, colonial durabilities can be interpreted as leaving selective spatial and, as I will explore in the next section, epistemic and atmospheric traces.

Atmospheric Antiblackness

Antiblack weather (Sharpe, 2016) is pervasive yet difficult to grasp and affects Black life in direct and indirect ways. In nineteenth- and early twentieth-century writings on disease, and meteorological weather in Sierra Leone the epistemic and antiblack entanglement of race, disease and place become apparent. Reading this section requires an understanding of the polysemy of the concepts of weather, climate and atmosphere. I refer to Sharpe's (2016) figurative use of weather to think through antiblackness in the wake as antiblack weather. But weather is also meteorological and, in the case of colonial disease control in Sierra Leone, weather, climate and atmospheres speak to histories of antiblack racism. In this section atmospheres denote two things: first, miasmata, the diseased airs and breezes that were thought to spread illness in the nineteenth and early twentieth century, and, second, affective atmospheres (Anderson, 2009), such as postcolonial spectres and hauntings (Coddington, 2011; cf. Bressey, 2014).

Race, Place, Disease

In what I am calling the weather, antiblackness is pervasive as climate. The weather necessitates changeability and improvisation; it is the atmospheric condition of time and place; it produces new ecologies. [...] The weather [transforms] Black being. [...] When the only certainty is the weather that produces a pervasive climate of antiblackness, what must we know in order to move through these environments in which the push is always toward Black death? (Sharpe, 2016, p. 106)

In nineteenth- and early twentieth-century scientific literature on Sierra Leone, weather, disease and antiblackness are closely linked. In the writings of white British scientists of the time, the Sierra Leonean weather *is* antiblack, not metaphorically, as is the case in Sharpe's writing, but by being presented as an agent through which Black African people could spread diseases to white Europeans. Their work also underlines the still contested fact, that science has always been political. One place in particular shaped English-speaking knowledge about Sierra Leone: the Liverpool School of Tropical Medicine. Shortly after its founding in 1899, the school sent its first (of many) expeditions to Sierra Leone to study the spread and prevalence of Malaria. Rubert Boyce (1863–1911), a pathologist and tropical disease expert and one of the school's members alongside Logan Taylor and Ronald Ross, dedicated his career to researching the origin and prevention of infectious, vector-borne diseases, most commonly appearing in the tropical regions of the British empire, such as West Africa and the West Indies as well as the southern US and South America. A considerable number of his publications draw on his expeditions to those regions and in the next and last chapters I analyse the link between colonial mobility and the constitution of infectious disease-related epistemology. Much more is known about Ronald Ross (Nye and Gibson, 1997), so I focus on Boyce's and Taylor's writings here instead.

In his book *Yellow Fever and Its Prevention: A Manual for Practitioners*, Boyce (1911a, p. 49) discusses yellow fever and malaria, two of the main diseases threatening the health of Europeans in West Africa as 'racial diseases' and their spread as a consequence of the transatlantic slave trade.

In the case of the sister disease, malaria, we do not discuss whether it was imported into West Africa or whether it was endemic. We regard it as a disease essentially endemic to those peoples living among Anophelines [mosquito transmitting malaria]. [...] In the eighteenth century the slave ship was no doubt one of the most powerful factors in the distribution, not only of yellow fever but of all other racial and endemic diseases and of the insect carriers peculiar to them. Not only did the slaveship [sic] carry human beings in whose blood might have been the virus of yellow fever, malaria, sleeping sickness, relapsing fever, filariasis, plague, etc – it equally well served as the means of transport of the various species of mosquitoes, fly, or flea. [...] The 'slaver' [slave ship] was a floating native village, in which the worst features of the native village were reproduced, white and blacks living jammed together in hot stifling quarters, providing the ideal conditions for the multiplication of the *Stegomyia* [a subgenus of the *Aedes aegypti*, the mosquito transmitting yellow fever] and the spread of yellow fever.

In an article published in the *British Medical Journal* in 1911 Boyce (1911b, p. 181) states 'as regards the West African continent [...] yellow fever was in all probability a disease endemial to the native races of the coast'. In his writings, yellow fever and malaria are associated with Blackness in two ways: they are anchored in Black places and bodies. Incidentally, during the preceding colonial period, Black colonial officers and troops were often selected for service in Sierra Leone because of their supposed tolerance for the West African climate and their ascribed immunity to diseases endemic to the region. The 'native village', in Boyce's writing, is depicted as the ideal breeding place for mosquitoes transmitting both diseases. Boyce (1910) points to the detrimental qualities of 'native' villages and how they are conducive to the spread of disease. Properties of place, in Boyce's writings, become attributes of the people living in those places. A lack of racial segregation and West African climatic conditions provide 'the ideal conditions for the multiplication of the *Stegomyia* and the spread of yellow fever' (Boyce, 1911a, p. 49). His reference to 'the worst features of the native village' also speaks to a perceived behavioural aspect of the spread of certain diseases. Antiblackness here is anchored in place and race. In Boyce's writing, the slave trade is only critiqued insofar as it led to the dissemination of infectious diseases across the British empire and, although captured Africans are described as human beings, their humanity is qualified by the conditions in which they choose (the native village) and are forced (the slave ship) to live.

Sierra Leone, from the beginning of Black and colonial settlements is, in Boyce's writing firmly imagined as a place of racialised disease. In this Boyce is not alone. In his writings he makes reference to other scientists who have contributed to a reading of Sierra Leone as a place of disease:

French writers have taken it for granted that Sierra Leone was the home of yellow fever on the West Coast, on the natural ground that it was more thickly peopled, and had wider relations with the outside world.

The origin of the [1835 yellow fever] outbreak was ascribed to importation from Fernando Po [Bioko, an island belonging to Equatorial Guinea], and by others to the town of Sangara, 400 miles distant. It was seriously proposed to build a high wall to keep out the pestilential breeze which, it was alleged, came from this town [Freetown]. (Boyce, 1911a, p. 181)

Freetown is imagined as a place of disease and as a place in which local atmospheres, people and the environment carry disease. At the same time, Freetown's forceful integration into the transatlantic economy is seen as having contributed to the spread of yellow fever. Boyce's reference to 'a pestilential breeze' (1911a, p. 181) is a reference to miasma theory. At Boyce's time of writing germ theory had replaced miasma theory as the acceptable rationale explaining the causes of disease. However, some of the authors Boyce (1910) draws on in his analysis made use of it.

When describing the history of yellow fever in Sierra Leone, Boyce (1911b) draws on Rankin's (1836) *The White Man's Grave: A Visit to Sierra Leone*. In one chapter, Rankin discusses the health and climate of Sierra Leone. Therein his references to infectious atmospheres and noxious weathers are frequent, as is his association of weather, atmosphere, disease and antiblackness.

An idea is extant that disease has originated in malaria brought thence by the north wind. When this idea was in vigour, various suggestions were offered for repelling the future intrusion of death from that quarter. [...] rather than detain the infectious air, [the natives] would rejoice in facilitating the greatest possible importation of it into the white man's settlement. (1836, pp. 147–8)

It is not easy therefore to discover in what manner or by what inlet the miasmata of the low country can enter to poison Sierra Leone. [...] Whatever detriments to health exist in Sierra Leone must arise from its own internal chemistry. (1836, p. 149)

As the only possible point of offence, these Maroon [resettled Jamaican maroons] grounds demand particular, if brief, notice. Noxious damps are considered to reach the European residences from it; [...] Assuming the origin of a foul atmosphere on this ground, Freetown has an advantage in its remote situation, and in the nature of the intervening space. (1836, p. 153)

In Rankin's writing, atmospheres, breezes and bad airs surround Black life in Sierra Leone and threaten the white colonial settler presence. The belief that diseases were caused and spread by bad airs are here inextricably linked to Sierra Leone as a diseased space. Miasma theory was equally applied in writings on Europe. In the case of Rankin's writings on Sierra Leone, however, these atmospheres are entangled with antiblackness.

In his writing (1836, pp. 147–8) 'the natives' 'rejoice' in threatening the health of white Europeans. The 'noxious damps' originating from 'Maroon grounds' also establish an epistemic link between Blackness, diseased atmospheres and place.

Boyce (1911a, p. 1) disavowed miasma theory and praised the onset of bacteriology and epidemiology. This scientific onset signals a shift in the relation between race, place and disease. While in Rankin's (1836) writings Black people were seen as living amidst unhealthy airs and constituting a threat to white health by propagating their spread to white settlements, Boyce (1910, p. 49) qualifies malaria and yellow fever as 'racial diseases'. Discussing endemicity, Boyce (1910) follows Sir Arthur Havelock, former governor of Sierra Leone, in discussing racial differences in yellow fever's infectious cycle. Boyce (1910, p. 58) quotes Havelock who, in 1884, sent a report on 'typho-malarial fever' to the Secretary of State as saying:[7] 'a noticeable feature was that as the disease assumed a more virulent type, it became more and more restricted to Europeans. The natives seemed to have complete immunity from its attacks, there not being a single authenticated case amongst the negro population.'

Boyce (1910, p. 62) added to this that '[t]he endemial remittent fever of the native was a source from which the *Stegomyia* [mosquito] obtained its infection'. Here scientific facts around malaria's endemicity in West Africa are used to deduce an understanding of Black people as diseased. The health threat they constitute to European settlers is also assessed. The endemic nature of malaria and yellow fever among Indigenous and resettled Black Sierra Leoneans was then used to justify the politics of sanitary segregation along racial lines in Freetown discussed above. In a paper on yellow fever in the *British Medical Journal*, Boyce (1911b, p. 181) argues that: 'If the mining managers and merchants will forearm themselves by adopting the rational precautions of segregation [...] they need not fear the awful setbacks to commercial progress [...].'

In a further shift, Logan Taylor, like Boyce a member of the Liverpool School of Tropical Medicine who conducted extensive sanitary work in Freetown, saw the behaviour of Sierra Leoneans more than the climate as the justification for racial segregation. He wrote (1902, pp. 853–4) that:

It is little wonder that Europeans and also natives living in the hot and damp West African climate, under conditions which favour the spread of malaria and other fevers, are taken ill, and it is these insanitary conditions more than purely climatic influences that are to blame for the unhealthiness of the West Coast. [...] Natives do not see the necessity for cleanliness, being quite content to remain as they are.

When suitable ground can be had I think it better for the Europeans to live away from the natives. In Accra the Government officials have good bungalows away from the native town, forming a proper European quarter (Victoriaborg), and this arrangement is found to work well, and Accra is the healthiest town on the Gold Coast. At Freetown a suitable site for a European quarter has been fixed on in the hills, and the proposed hill railway to it has been already surveyed.

The widespread support for sanitary segregation on racial grounds is evident in Taylor's writings and in their being published in the *British Medical Journal*. These writings also showcase that the association of disease and place was, in the case of colonial Sierra Leone, still characterised by antiblackness. The causes of the 'unhealthiness' of Sierra Leone are here linked to both the local meteorological climate and to the behaviour of 'natives'. As a consequence, only spatial distance from Black people and grounds can protect European settlers from infection.

In the case of infectious diseases and their prevention in Sierra Leone, the perception of diseased atmospheres and antiblackness combined to inform sanitary segregation policies in Freetown. With regard to Sierra Leone, knowledge of infectious diseases and infectious disease control has long been characterised by epistemic antiblackness. In the scientific texts the speculated relation between Blackness and disease is threefold: first, disease stems from 'native grounds' and is spread through bad airs; second, Sierra Leone's climate and environment is one in which 'racial diseases' are endemic; and, finally, the insanitary behaviour of the native Black population produces and spreads disease. This epistemic antiblackness contributed to the imagination of Sierra Leone as a place of disease and danger for white colonisers. During the Ebola epidemic, the idea of Sierra Leone as a place of disease and as a place which threatened white European health was reaffirmed.

The Weather

International responders to the Ebola virus outbreak in Sierra Leone also found themselves in what they encountered as challenging climatic conditions. Meteorological weather featured in several interviews with international doctors and nurses who deployed to Sierra Leone to work against the spread of Ebola virus, and almost always in relation to their capacity to care or not care for African Ebola patients. Weather conditions varied according to treatment centres, with the majority of British-based international health workers working in purpose-built ETCs, which were generally hotter than pre-existing brick facilities. A lack of qualified doctors and treatment beds prior to the outbreak (WHO, 2015; Global Fund, 2017; Tinsley, 2018) constituted one major reason for the construction of purpose-built ETCs, a majority of which were tent-structures, which afforded little protection from the sun and heat of Sierra Leone's weather.

British colonial health and sanitation policy 'was largely designed to meet the needs of the white, expatriate community' (Cole, 2014, p. 239). As such, few efforts were made to sustainably cater for the health of the colony beyond its white settlers (Cole, 2014). Despite British parasitologist and tropical disease specialist Ronald Ross's (Anonymous, 1901) urging to sustainably improve Freetown's health conditions by draining its streets and swamps to reduce breeding grounds for mosquitoes (work undertaken in the following years by Logan Taylor), thereby lowering the risk of malaria for all residents, the colonial government opted primarily for racial sanitary segregation instead.[8] Sanitary segregation had the added benefit of conveying a sense of biological difference to support a claim to cultural superiority shared by many white European settlers. One of the reasons for not investing in sustainable health care in Freetown was the transitory nature of colonial officers, who only stayed for a short number of years before returning to the UK (Spitzer, 1968). Eventually however, to make the West African colonies 'healthier' and attract a bigger medical work force, the West African Medical Service (WAMS) was created in 1901 and tasked with supplying medical doctors to serve in the six West African colonies. The WAMS formally excluded Black West African doctors from applying, making it one of the first openly racially segregated UK government departments of the twentieth century (Johnson, 2010).

As a result of racist recruitment and health and sanitation policies, 'native' health and well-being, especially outside of Freetown, was drastically underfunded (Cole, 2014). 'Native' Freetown and the West African coast more generally were seen as detrimental to European health in virtue of their racial and environmental constitution rather than as a result of colonial policies that considered Black health as at once irrelevant and threatening to white settlers. Due to the absence of medical facilities of the kind available in the 'European' section of the town and meteorological conditions that British settlers and scientists considered toxic, Black health was only minimally cared for and the risk of death from diseases was high (Cole, 2014). British colonial policy laid the groundwork for an underfunded health infrastructure, both in terms of not training medical staff and a dearth of places of care, and as Frankfurter et al. (2019) have shown, by relying on *indirect rule*, to govern the Sierra Leone Protectorate.

In 2014, the lack of permanent healthcare facilities, combined with insufficient numbers of trained Sierra Leonean medical staff to respond to the epidemic, created another kind of antiblack climate, in which conditions would once again be experienced as dangerous for international personnel. While lacking the openly racist framing of the colonial period, the 2014–16 response was enacted in conditions that were reminiscent of the groundwork laid in the colonial period and thereby continued to be entangled with antiblackness.

The weather, as it was described by international health workers who worked in the international Ebola response in Sierra Leone, impacted working conditions in Ebola treatment centres. In Sierra Leone day-time temperatures vary between 26°C and 36°C (Blinker, 2006). The healthcare workers I interviewed worked either in purpose-built ETCs or in pre-existing facilities that were adapted to constitute safe working environments and serve the purposes of isolating sick patients. Both types of facilities were impacted by Sierra Leonean weather. For Ebola, which at the time had no proven cure, the best method of treatment was aggressive rehydration through the administration of either ORS (oral rehydration solution) or IV (intravenous therapy) (Farmer, 2014). The time required to administer as many of these treatments as possible became a crucial factor in treating EVD and the weather played an important role in health care workers' ability to care for patients. Charlotte, a British nurse who worked in a new purpose-built ETC, described the weather and working conditions in the following way:

> It was brimming hot when we were there. Hot and humid. It was the hottest time of the year, so yeah, I spent relatively little time in the red zone of all the time I was out there. [...] We were there at the hottest time of the year, so [...] only at night could you be in there for longer, but during the day we were only allowed to be in the red zone for 40 minutes. [...] If people are hot and if you need to go you need to go, so you're halfway through a job and you just left it on the side.

The red zone in ETCs was the area of the hospital or treatment centre in which confirmed, and in some instances suspect, cases awaited results. In order to enter the red zone, health care workers had to wear full personal protective equipment (PPE). PPE was put on or 'donned' according to strict rules and involved several layers of protective equipment to avoid potentially contagious bodily fluids from being transmitted from patients to carers. Charlotte described the process thus:

> You would start with one pair of gloves and then you would go and take off your outer stuff, your normal clothes, wash your hands to start with and then you would put on your suit and you would put on your mask first or hood first, we had slightly different PPE to the others but then you'd put your outer gloves [...] but you're sweating by the time you've put it on you know, so then it's this very ritualistic, ordered thing [...].

The impenetrability of PPE contributed to making the hot temperatures even less bearable. Gareth, an infectious disease specialist who worked in a hospital in Freetown, a pre-existing adapted brick facility, compared the work he had to do there, to occasions on which he had to work in a purpose-built facility, in this case a tent:

> The tents were incredibly hot. Phenomenally hot. [...] I have an image of a meeting in a tent and everyone was wearing PPE and you can just see one of the army guys in uniform and they're just drenched all the way through, because the tent was actually baking. And [...] when you're working in a brick environment it's actually reasonably cool. [...] I think generally when we went in to do the work in the unit, we'd be in there for about two to three hours and that was reasonably comfortable.

According to Gareth, working in a brick environment made the heat and working in PPE more bearable. Unlike those who worked in a tent-like purpose-built facility, like Charlotte, health care workers in brick units could stay in PPE for up to three hours. Pre-existing, durable units thus seemed to allow health care workers to provide longer and more thorough care for patients in the hot weather. Alex, a South African doctor, worked in the same facility as Gareth and described the sensation of wearing PPE in the heat:

In these crazy suits, it's really really fucking hot, like you can only be in there for a certain time because otherwise you actually physiologically can't sustain it. Some people handle heat better than me. I found the heat that was the most difficult part. You get to the end and your boots are filled with water and you're not sure what it is. Is it your own sweat, did you spill something on yourself? [laughs] What is this sensation of water in your gumboots? What's going on? So yeah it was very hard and difficult.

Alex's statement illustrates both the constraints meteorological weather exerted on the organisation of care work during the Ebola epidemic as well as the emotional toll it took on both care workers and patients. Although they laughed when recounting the sensation of working in PPE in hot conditions, they continued to describe the oppressive atmosphere for patients to which the heat, in their opinion, contributed: 'It's a terrifying scenario to be in, 'cause it's really hot, there's these people in big white suits coming at you, no one is really talking to you, you don't know what's happening, people around you are dying.'

Hot weather and the high contagiousness of EVD in combination with a lack of adequate medical infrastructure contributed to affective atmospheres of fear and stress. The weather did play a role in how, and how much, care could be administered with pre-existing brick facilities allowing health care workers to stay in the unit in full PPE for longer. During the epidemic, the weather had little to do with the antiblackness or antiblack weather (Sharpe, 2016) that has shaped Sierra Leone's healthcare system since colonial times. However, the historical lack of investment in medical care for all Sierra Leoneans and the structural underfunding that resulted from it, led to safe medical care predominantly being located in purpose-built ETCs. In these ETCs, tents for the most part, weather conditions made caring for Sierra Leonean patients much more difficult than in pre-existing brick facilities.

During colonialism, Black health was mostly seen in terms of its potential to harm white settler colonisers and, consequently, little attention was paid to Black health and to the structural foundations that would ensure that the latter was in good condition. Racially segregated health facilities and medical racism have left their trace on Freetown in material form. This had repercussions on the conditions in which the Ebola response could operate. The limited availability of suitable pre-existing medical facilities in which patients could be isolated directly impacted the possibilities to care for and save Black lives.

Atmospheres of (Colonial) Haunting

I finish this chapter by writing about affective atmospheres (Anderson, 2009) and affective hospital infrastructures (Street, 2011, 2014) and specifically about affective atmospheres that border on hauntings and spectres. I suggest that places of care, during the Ebola epidemic were also places of colonial and antiblack haunting. I suggest that in Sierra Leone the wake encompasses more than the physical remains of slavery and colonialism, and that the rumours around places of care, which abounded during the epidemic, can be interpreted as a processing of past antiblack violence that occurred here, but which has left no tangible trace. As Richardson et al. (2019, p. 1) have argued in the context of the EVD outbreak in the Democratic Republic of Congo (DRC) (2018–19), studies on rumours or mistrust often 'inadvertently relegate consideration of the historical antecedents of [Congolese] "lack of trust" to outside the domain of "valid" public health research, consideration and action'. This book adopts a different approach. Here, studying places of care in the wake relies on a sense of place attuned to the antiblack practices and discourses that have shaped care in relation to Sierra Leonean life, enslaved, colonised and free, in Freetown. Here I focus on fears and rumours around Ebola's origins and its supposed political purpose and its association with places and practices of care.

Luise White's (2000) historical exploration of East African rumours and vampire stories locates their origin in colonial medical practices, such as forced trials or medical experiments. Relying on archival sources and oral histories, White (2000, pp. 106–7) describes a Kenyan woman who in 1920s Nairobi related the violence of Kenyan encounters with medical practitioners: '[they] used to come in the night, they would come into your room very softly and before you knew it they put something in your arm to draw out the blood. [...] Medical practitioners come to Africans, unannounced and unwelcomed, and do not heal, but silence and kill.'

Similar concerns abounded during the Sierra Leonean Ebola epidemic. During the epidemic, white Western biomedicine became a force regulating the lives and deaths of Freetonians (Lipton, 2017). Lipton describes (2017, p. 808) 'the imposing presence of the novel biomedical order honed to eliminate the virus' and argues that this biomedical order, characterised by standardised, non-traditional, impersonal burials, was perceived as white. Several writers (Richards, 2016; Spencer, 2015; Lipton, 2017) have described the importance of traditional burials in Sierra Leone, which are seen to ensure the well-being of deceased relatives in the afterlife. White biomedicine disrupted these practices and endangered the 'deceased's eternal fate' (Lipton, 2017, p. 808). Seeking care in a hospital equalled subjecting oneself to white biomedicine and the perceived risks associated with biomedical care, such as non-traditional burials, risking one's eternal fate and a form of violence that mirrors White's (2000) accounts.

Interviews with Sierra Leonean and international responders revealed that many Ebola patients were reluctant to seek help in internationally run treatment centres. This was confirmed by media reports. In a BBC interview broadcast on 1 August 2014, Dr Oliver Johnson, a British doctor standing in front of the isolation unit at Connaught Hospital, stated: 'There's fear and concern among the patients who either don't believe that the disease is real or don't trust the hospitals to treat them. So they're staying away from the hospital, they're refusing to be isolated here' (BBC, 2014).

The fear and concern that Dr Johnson describes found expression in rumours. Here, I treat rumours that circulated around medical care and care places as a representation of past experience and a way of processing present events through that past. The reluctance to seek care in 'white' treatment centres is indicative of the wake and its geographies, and an analysis of the latter can offer insights into places of care and medical responses in postcolonial contexts. Following Coddington (2011, pp. 146–7), I take hauntings as 'aspects of social life which appear to be not there, concealed yet important; aspects which *seethe, acting on* or *meddling with* present-day realities in a violent or disturbed manner; and finally, aspects that by seething, unsettle taken-for-granted realities'. These hauntings, like weather, are at once present and at times hard to notice. I suggest that hauntings, rather than appearing to Sierra Leoneans but not international health workers, emerge between the two and shape and unsettle their relationship with regard to Ebola care.

The Ebola epidemic spread from the border region of south-eastern Guinea to Sierra Leone and Liberia in the first half of 2014 and by 1 August the first Ebola cases were reported in Freetown. As Dr Johnson told the BBC, patients were reluctant to be treated in hospitals and treatment centres. The healthcare responders I interviewed confirmed facing similar problems when working in ETCs around the country. Anne, a British nurse who worked as the clinical lead in an ETC outside of Freetown, talked about patients' reluctance to visit their facility: 'they were a very resisting community, like lots of rumours. It was challenging for our psychosocial team to work with the community there, for people to accept to come to Ebola treatment centres and they were often hiding sick people.'

From a biomedical standpoint, what was at stake was convincing Sierra Leoneans suspected of carrying the virus to come to hospitals or treatment centres. Anne's statement that 'they were a very resisting community' and that 'they were often hiding sick people' indicates that, rather than seeking medical care in their vicinity, some Sierra Leoneans tried to put individuals infected with the Ebola virus outside of the reach of biomedical care and the clinic. Emmanuel, a Sierra Leonean nurse, worked for an international organisation in Sierra Leone during the epidemic. He explained that:

> there was a lot of conspiracy theory about how Ebola was spread, so the local people did not have any confidence in international organisations. So because of that lack of trust, we needed to convince people that this was a medical response, it wasn't political, you know there was no ulterior motive.

Conspiracy theories and rumours were a sign of mistrust in international organisations. This mistrust extended to places of biomedical care and was based in historical conflations of violent, often extractive, medical praxis and health care sites. Anton, who worked at Connaught Hospital, related a common rumour: 'I heard rumours about people getting killed in those places [hospitals and ETCs] or that it was all a big conspiracy, but considering the availability of information and the sort of context I am not gonna say they're unreasonable.'

Like Anton, some responders were aware that relations between hospitals and local communities during the Ebola epidemic were fraught with tension and mistrust from the start. Patients did not trust the hospital as a place in which to receive care. This mistrust constitutes an instance of postcolonial haunting. Historically, (white) biomedicine and antiblack violence coincided in Sierra Leone in places of care. This historical relationship 'meddl[ed] with present-day realities' (Coddington, 2011, p. 147) in a way that shaped the ability of international health workers to care for Sierra Leonean lives during the Ebola response. Anne's statements mirrored Anton's descriptions of mistrust. When describing the spraying of chlorine for disinfection purposes she told me that: 'Some people would think you were trying to kill them essentially. 'Cause they can report that to their family and say "they're trying to gas us". That was one of the fears with the spraying of chlorine when people were getting into ambulances. [It's] like you're being gassed basically. [...] [That was] a rumour point.'

Like Anton and Anne, James, a British doctor described the rumours related to Connaught hospital in which he worked and their consequences for national and international health workers, working in the Ebola unit:

A lot of our early problems were not so much that Ebola was a curse, not a virus, it was that Ebola was a conspiracy. So there was a belief that we were taking patients into the unit to kill them, inject them to kill them or there was another belief, I read a quote from someone, [...] who [...] talks about how, his belief before he got sick was that they wanted our blood, people who didn't have blood had come to take his blood. And when he got sick a nurse he had known from his community for many years treated him in the Ebola unit and [...] rather than believing her he simply believed that she had been kind of co-opted and they'd come to take his blood and you know that must have been September/October [2014] time.

This shows that between White's (2000) research in East and Central Africa and the Ebola outbreak in Sierra Leone, rumours remained consistent in their content and in relation to the same practice (drawing blood). While there is no way of directly linking these rumours back to colonial biomedical practice, they can be interpreted as resulting from similar colonial histories. James's account also indicates how deeply entrenched and resistant these beliefs were ('rather than believing her he simply believed she had been co-opted'). His statement illustrates that, rather than being solely a medical phenomenon, Ebola, the environment in which it took place and the practices necessary for medical care were a social phenomenon haunted by the colonial and antiblack past. This had repercussions for patients' readiness to seek care from international (and predominantly white) healthcare workers and to seek help in places of care that were associated with (white) biomedicine. James continued:

Certainly, in the early time, there was unrest, patients were trying to escape, family members were trying to break their family members out [...] soldiers were deployed to our unit, there was a big question around should we forcibly restrain patients from leaving? Patients were very unlikely to be referred, you know they didn't want to come [...] And we had families, rioting [in] the hospital believing that Ebola was a conspiracy intended for us to kill their family member. You know Dr X once was chased up the stairs by family members and she locked herself in our office with us and we were worried they might set the building on fire. It was quite a real challenge and you know the idea of physical harm became quite real.

Here hauntings, and the antiblack past they evoke, shape postcolonial presents and biomedical environments. Rumours provide discursive anchoring for haunting atmospheres. The colonial past haunts present biomedical reality and lived possibilities for Black life and health in Sierra Leone. This haunting, although it often occurs in relation to colonial medicine, both epistemically and spatially, is difficult to grasp and almost impossible to pin down. When considered in relation to existing literature on rumours, haunting and colonial medicine (White, 2000; Coddington, 2011), however, the importance of recognising these spectres of colonial medicine and the violence that characterised it, become clear. The violence of the slave trade has left its marks on the Sierra Leonean landscape and is remembered in cultural and mundane practices (Ferme, 2001; Shaw, 2002). During the Ebola epidemic those memories materialised in rumours and hauntings surrounding places of (white) biomedical care.

Conclusion

The colonial wake, in which the Ebola epidemic took place, manifests in more or less conspicuous remains. Today, life in Sierra Leone is itself in the wake of the Ebola epidemic. According to one interviewee, being in the wake of Ebola also gave rise to a sense of haunting. Rather than a postcolonial haunting, the place of care that this responder described was haunted by the epidemic itself. Charlotte, a British nurse, was part of the last deployment that was sent out by the NHS to Sierra Leone in January 2015. She worked in one of the purpose-built ETCs erected by the British and Sierra Leonean armies to cope with high numbers of infections at the height of the epidemic. Charlotte describes the treatment centre when the last patient left:

One of the most surreal experiences was actually when they shut, when the last survivors left and [...] I think I was on the shift or some of us volunteered and we went in and sorted it out, because it was chaos in there, because people go in and you know everything that goes in can't come out so you had just like chaos of stuff and rubbish [...] and being in the red zone without patients and I really felt that from some of the staff, it was like the ghosts of the people that had died there then rose up to meet [you], like you could then process it because you weren't in there looking after patients, you were ... yeah the red zone without patients in it, it's a very very odd and ghostly place. And it felt haunted, it really did feel haunted [...].

Charlotte's account interrogates places of care and their remains, and how these places influence the relationship between patients, health care workers and medical care. Like the ways in which colonial medical practices have left their traces on the development of the Ebola epidemic and the possibilities of care within the response, the epidemic itself will likely haunt, positively or negatively, future relations between Sierra Leoneans, medical interventions and the places in which care is provided.

Hauntings, like the weather, like affective atmospheres, like the wake, are not always immediately tangible or visible. Antiblackness, like meteorological weather, shifts and circulates and, depending on one's perspective and experience, is more or less conspicuous. Both require a sensitivity towards the pervasiveness of colonial and antiblack violence and the tenacity of colonial space-making. The wake, and the antiblackness that characterises it, assume various forms – material, epistemic or atmospheric – and are present in and through places, spaces and practices. They hold the possibilities in which Black Sierra Leonean life exists today and came sharply into focus during the Ebola epidemic, many aspects of which were reminiscent of Sierra Leone's colonial past.

2

Colonial Mobilities and Infrastructures: The Production of (Anti)Blackness

Introduction

> For three weary days our gallant ship had apparently become aware of its approach towards an evil shore. No longer cutting a rapid and gay path through legions of waves, she had lingered as if reluctant to bear her crew to the land of pestilence and death. (F. Harrison Rankin, 1836, p. 1)

He is setting out for England on a ship. She has a letter with an address written on it, a place in London where an uncle lives. That's where she will go. He is excited and scared and hopeful and –. The ship becomes a plane and then reverts back to being a ship. It takes Mary Kingsley 14 days to travel from Liverpool to Sierra Leone. It takes Aminata six and a half hours to travel from London to Freetown. It takes me 13. People embark on voyages in England. They board planes in London. They set sail from Liverpool. People are herded onto ships in Sierra Leone, unwillingly. People leave from England, from Nova Scotia, from Jamaica, full of hope. Years pass, nothing changes. Everything changes. Nobody had told him he was Black until he tried to board. Until he tried to leave. Always to come back here, to Sierra Leone, but they don't let him. Leave that is, so that she can come back. So that they can come back. Journeys make places and people and unmake them in turn. They also make Blackness.

The Ebola epidemic and response revealed dynamics that have long been at the heart of colonialism and enslavement: the regulation and politics of Black mobilities. In this chapter I think through transatlantic mobilities and the production of Blackness, and specifically about how the mobilities linking Sierra Leone and the United Kingdom produce Blackness in reference to a colonial-racial hierarchy that holds both places and the mobilities that link them.[1] I draw on Achille Mbembe's (2017, p. 30) work, which points to the importance of various mobilities (slave trade, colonialism, Black migration and travel to Europe and Africa) in the development of both 'Western' and 'Black' consciousnesses of Blackness, and the importance of mobilities in the making of 'the modern Black imaginary': 'Ideas circulated within a vast global network, producing the modern Black imaginary. The creators of the imaginary were often people in motion, crossing constantly from one continent to another.'

The mobilities that link Sierra Leone and the UK reveal their entanglements with the production of Blackness. These build on enduring infrastructures that signal colonial continuity and the colonial wake in which the Ebola response took place. Building on Mimi Sheller's (2018) definition of 'mobility injustice' as 'the process through which unequal spatial conditions and differential subjects are made', I show that the British-led international response to the Sierra Leonean Ebola outbreak constitutes a site of colonial-racial 'mobility injustice'. I extend her work to show that the Ebola epidemic and response exacerbated and exhibited a process in which the mobilities that contributed to the making of unequal spatial conditions were linked to the production of Blackness. In this chapter I focus on antiblackness and infrastructure and antiblackness *as* infrastructure.

Blackness is not a monolith. 'Racial boundaries are formed, reformed and transformed through mobile relations of power' (Sheller, 2018, p. 57). I suggest here that the mobilities linking Sierra Leone and the UK, and their regulation, allow the tracing of various perceptions of Blackness as produced through the transatlantic slave trade, British colonialism, Sierra Leonean independence and the Ebola epidemic. The Ebola epidemic and response forces us to think through the long-standing tensions at the heart of what I call a 'Black mobile ontology'.[2] Mobilities are a central factor in the production of Blackness as the 'ontological negation of being' (Sharpe, 2016, p. 14) through commodification, subjection, criminalisation and in the case of the Ebola epidemic, disease and death. At the same time mobilities also contribute to the making of Black diasporic ontologies as mobile, sovereign selves. The contemporary infrastructures that underlie these mobilities are evocative of Sierra Leone's colonial past and the colonial-racial hierarchies that shaped it. By analysing mobilities and the production of Blackness I develop a theme that Black Studies evokes but does not explicitly address in relation to colonial Africa. Analyses of Black (im)mobilities have for the most part occurred within the context of the US and the Caribbean. In those analyses, West Africa is conceptualised as being linked to contemporary mobilities only through its existence in the distant past.

In this chapter, as in the book more generally, I move between the past and the present. Between theory and empirics. There are more straightforward ways of telling stories, but bear with me. There is method to my movement. In taking the roundabout way, in revisiting the past time and again, we insist on its nowness; its circularity (Olufemi, 2021). This circularity characterises Black experiences. Often being caught by the past, having the same thing happen again and again. And again. This can feel and read as tedious. Black mobilities too, are often shaped by the frequent reminder that, as much as we move in the here and now, our movements are shaped by past perceptions and, at times, by future impossibility; that they are held back. So, I issue an invitation: let us think through a Black mobile ontology together, the roundabout way. Antiblackness hides in the places we pass by when taking the straightforward way. This can be tedious, but it is a move towards justice.

In the wake, Sierra Leone exists as multiple places and has multiple mobile ontologies (Sheller, 2018), which depend on the existence and framing of British–Sierra Leonean mobilities and infrastructures. Following Patricia Noxolo (2006, p. 265) I formulate an analysis of these ontologies that depends on a critical geography of Sierra Leone as a place 'that comprises all the places that have contributed and continue to contribute to its history and culture'. The flows connecting Sierra Leone to the UK are the ones I focus on here. One might argue that they play a particularly important role in this geography. On the other hand, centring them also reinscribes their importance in the narratives that shape Sierra Leone in the present. I do so here, to take them apart. The chapter focuses on maritime and aerial mobilities. Aerial transport technologies, such as planes or helicopters became highly relevant during the Ebola outbreak because of the apparent threat their speed and global connectivity posed to the containment of viral agents. The threat of the spread of disease was most often associated with infected aeroplane passengers coming from Sierra Leone, Liberia and Guinea. All accidental introductions of EVD into Western countries involved flights carrying infected passengers from affected West African countries into Europe and via Europe into the United States.

I start in the past, with an analysis of historical British–Sierra Leonean mobilities. Here, I take routes, directionality, and material and human infrastructure as three instances to analyse how, during the transatlantic slave trade, colonialism and the moment of independence, mobilities linking the UK and Sierra Leone produced Blackness as absence, deviance and dependence.[3] In the process, whiteness, without being named, is predominantly produced as antithetical to Blackness and white and Black spaces are framed and shaped differently through these mobilities. The second part of the chapter looks at contemporary mobilities and the making of diasporic and Sierra Leonean mobile ontologies. Postcolonial mobile ontologies, both of people and places, are still produced in relation to the UK as colonial centre, a phenomenon which was exacerbated during and after the Ebola epidemic and response. The suspension of direct flights between Sierra Leone and the UK at the moment of the Ebola epidemic not only shows the entanglement of modern diasporic lives with what Mbembe (2017) calls 'Western consciousness of Blackness', but also the Black diasporic production of Sierra Leone as a place of opportunity, or what Mbembe (2017) defines as an aspect of 'Black consciousness of Blackness'.

Overall, for Black Sierra Leoneans and white British colonial/contemporary responders, mobilities between the two countries have always been different and have construed the country and themselves as different people and places. The loss felt by the Sierra Leonean community in the UK when faced with the discontinuation of direct flights needs to be seen as part of a long history of Black immobilisation and mobile disruption. From the British point of view, economic profit calculations always underlay mobilities to and from Sierra Leone, whereas for Sierra Leoneans they came to be an expression of a privileged postcolonial relationship with the former colonial centre.

Colonial Mobilities and Infrastructures

Here I analyse the colonial entanglements of Sierra Leonean–British mobilities. I consider the establishment of routes, regulations and infrastructures as suggestive of the shifting production of Blackness. By looking at present-day airline routes I briefly argue that the way in which transatlantic mobilities currently play out is based on a disregard for the commodification of Black life at the very heart of the establishment of transatlantic mobilities. Further, I suggest that this disregard frames British colonial mobilities towards Sierra Leone as mobilities of care, rather than exploitation, contributing to the erasure of white supremacist violence and working towards white innocence. Commercial aeromobilities into Sierra Leone were part and parcel of the colonial enterprise and white mobilities into the empire were implicitly encouraged and normalised, whereas Black mobilities towards the UK were explicitly discouraged and criminalised. This differentiation is evocative of the production of Blackness as deviance and risk, whose circulation colonial governance aimed to control. Finally, I analyse human and material colonial infrastructures, with the latter referring to the built environment and show that these were in part designed to guarantee continued British access to Sierra Leonean resources after independence. This signals the colonial wake.

The Establishment of Routes

Current aeromobilities are built on a history of transport mobilities that disregards Black mobilities and the violence of early transatlantic population flows. This disregard can offer a possible explanation for current passenger aeromobilities which largely leave Africa off the map. An analysis of available airline routes in the late 2000s showed that flight connections were densest between Europe and North America (Jpatokal, 2009). Less dense are the flight connections linking Africa, and West Africa in particular, to the world, indicating a scarcity of routes. Eric Sheppard (2002, p. 319) explains this disconnect historically by arguing that early efforts to connect London with New York were first enhanced through transport technologies, the steamship, the aeroplane or the telegraph, along routes on which 'large shares of commodities and information already flowed'. He contrasts this example with that of 'major African cities' (Sheppard, 2002, p. 319), which are still poorly connected both to each other and to European hubs. His analysis suggests that African cities were disconnected from the flow of commodities and capital he describes. Sheppard's (2002) analysis leaves out the role the trade in African lives played in establishing modern capital and transport flows across the Atlantic.

For 400 years the slave trade shaped the transatlantic region, connecting Africa's western coast to Europe and the Americas (and in the case of the Indian Ocean slave trade, its eastern coast). According to the Trans-Atlantic Slave Trade Database (2013) 33,822 voyages were made on ships transporting close to 10 million enslaved Africans across the Atlantic. As Mbembe (2017, p. 14) has pointed out '[b]etween 1630 and 1780, far more Africans than Europeans disembarked in Great Britain's Atlantic colonies.' Despite the total volume of journeys, ships, enslaved and cargo transported from West Africa across the Atlantic, West Africa today scarcely features on a global map of transatlantic flight connections. Taking contemporary transport mobilities to be anchored in historical capitalist flows also marginalises the considerable wealth generated by European and North American individuals and nations through the slave trade. Money from the slave trade contributed to the establishment of British banks, universities and private fortunes, and significantly enriched British Victorian cities such as London, Bristol or Liverpool (Hall et al., 2014). However, in the subsequent establishment of transatlantic passenger and cargo shipping, telegraph and aeroplane routes, Africa was largely left off the map. Consequently, early transatlantic flows manifested for the Black populations of Africa as violent extractive mobilities while founding the wealth which built contemporary transport mobilities. In the present, African lives are still largely left off this map. This disparity is indicative of the racial-colonial 'mobility injustice' (Sheller, 2018) in which the Ebola epidemic took place.

Both the UK and Sierra Leone constituted major regions involved in the transatlantic slave trade (Trans-Atlantic Slave Trade Database, 2013). Ships from the UK, in particular from London, Bristol and Liverpool ports, carried 34.2 per cent of all enslaved people across the Atlantic. Approximately 12,000 slave voyages were undertaken by ships sailing under British flags and Sierra Leone was the principal place of slave purchase on 1,153 voyages.

During the time of the slave trade, Sierra Leone became a geographical hub of importance at least twice, first in becoming a location from and via which enslaved Africans were shipped on European vessels from sub-Saharan Africa to North and South America and the Caribbean, thus enhancing transport mobilities both in terms of establishing naval routes and the infrastructures required for maritime navigation (see Figure 9).

The second time Sierra Leone became a geographical hub was in disrupting these very routes and mobilities, after the abolition of the British slave trade, when slave ships were stopped by the British Navy and returned to Sierra Leone, the nearest British port, to be tried in the Court of Mixed Commissions, which could potentially lead to the freeing of recaptured slaves (Fyfe, 1962; Martinez, 2012; Olusoga, 2016). With regard to the transatlantic slave trade in Sierra Leone, ships became a metaphor of both violence and liberation.

This liberation framed Sierra Leone's subsequent colonisation by the British Crown as an act of care. In the remains of King's Yard Gate, Brit-

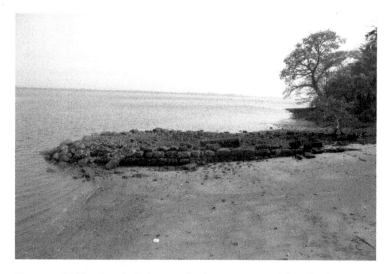

Figure 9   Old landing dock, Bunce Island, Sierra Leone. (Photo by the author)
Bunce Island was the site of an important slave-trading post. Its location in
the Sierra Leone River made it accessible for slave ships. Enslaved Africans
were transported to Bunce from Sierra Leone's mainland on smaller
boats before being shipped across the Atlantic. Conservation efforts were
undertaken between 2017 and 2020 to preserve Bunce Island's slave-trading
infrastructures.

ain's hand in the commodification of Blackness is erased and what remains
are reminders of mobilities of care. Both flows shaped Sierra Leone to differing degrees. The contemporary disregard for the Black mobilities that
both fuelled early capitalism and produced Blackness as an 'ontological negation of being' (Sharpe, 2016, p. 14) by turning Black bodies into
'*bodies of extraction*' (Mbembe, 2017), necessitates a reading of present-day
mobilities in which Blackness is absent or dependent. This mobility injustice is indicative of being immobilised and left off the map, of Blackness
as marginal to the flows of capital and power. This marginalisation plays
an important role in the aftermath of the Ebola epidemic. A closer look at
colonial mobility regulations lays the basis for my analysis of contemporary UK–Sierra Leone mobilities during the 2014–16 Ebola epidemic that
I attend to in the second part of this chapter.

Colonial Mobilities: Directionality

The production of Blackness as deviant and risky can be observed in the
differential framing of directionality between Sierra Leone and the UK.

Mbembe (2017, p. 35) argues that 'race is what makes it possible to identify and define population groups in a way that makes each of them carriers of differentiated and more or less shifting risk'. During British colonialism, predominantly white mobilities from the UK to Sierra Leone were encouraged, blurring the line between colonial officers and British civilians, whereas Black Sierra Leonean mobilities towards the UK were discouraged, producing Black Sierra Leoneans as risky subjects and criminalising their movements. The mobilities linking the two countries have thus long been entangled with the production of racial difference. The regulation of mobilities and the politicisation of directionality shaped constructions of Britain and Sierra Leone as colonial centre and dependent respectively. These dynamics extend into the present, shape Black Sierra Leonean mobility, and impacted the international Ebola response in Sierra Leone. Sierra Leone's status as colony was reified and upheld through a regulation of its people's mobilities. It is not only Sierra Leone as a place that was colonised, but Sierra Leonean mobilities too, in that they were imbued with colonial-racial hierarchies. Stoler (2016, p. 117) offers a definition of colonies that places the regulation of mobilities at its very centre:

A 'colony' as a common noun is a place where people are moved in and out; a place of livid, hopeful, desperate, and violent circulation. [...] A 'colony' as a political concept is not a place but a principle of managed mobilities, mobilizing and immobilizing populations according to a set of changing rules, for resettlement, for disposal, for aid, or for coerced labour and those who are forcibly confined.

Stoler's (2016) definition is useful in that it draws attention to several aspects which are reflected and can be traced in the history of colonial mobility regulation in Sierra Leone. In her writing the colony is defined as a place of violent circulation. For several hundred years Sierra Leone was a place of violent antiblack circulation. I now turn to its nature as colony and specifically to colonial Sierra Leone as 'a principle of managed mobilities' (Stoler, 2016, p. 117). Speaking of Sierra Leone in that sense allows for an analysis of how colonialism, through the regulation of mobilities, laid the basis for the relatively free global mobility afforded to predominantly white European and North American citizens compared to the relative immobility of (predominantly Brown and Black) former colonial subjects. This racial differentiation became visible during the Ebola outbreak. How the colonial management of mobilities intersected with the management of infectious diseases historically is the subject of the following section.

The material, human and epistemological flows linking Freetown to London have always been subject to different rules and regulations from those linking London with Freetown and have shaped the respective cities to differing degrees in terms of domination/immersion. Mobilities towards Sierra Leone and within British West Africa were actively encouraged, at least for colonial officers. The coordination of medical and sanitary policies relied actively on these intercolonial and inter-imperial mobilities, first undertaken by ship and later by plane. After the onset of a yellow fever outbreak in Freetown in 1913, Rubert Boyce, an infectious and tropical diseases expert, was summoned from England. A Yellow Fever Report (Wellcome Trust, GC/59/A), written for the West African Yellow Fever Commission in 1913 describes his arrival as follows:

> Sir Rubert Boyce, who had sailed from England on June 1st with additional medical officers to render assistance in the Gold Coast and Sierra Leone, arrived at Freetown on his outward journey to Secondee about June 13th, a few days after the death of a European (Case 11) from Yellow Fever. After consultation with the Senior Sanitary Officer, he decided to continue his journey to Secondee, leaving behind him two of the medical officers to assist in carrying out the preventive measures. Quarantine was raised from Freetown at the end of June, all necessary anti-mosquito measures being continued.

West African intercolonial and British–Sierra Leonean mobility was seen as instrumental for the coordination of infectious disease control in Sierra Leone. Boyce's journey from England also indicates that, according to British decision makers, the knowledge and expertise deemed necessary to combat the yellow fever outbreak did not exist locally but had to be summoned from the UK, a point I return to in the chapter on expertise (chapter 4). As with the liberation of freed slaves, these mobilities framed British–Sierra Leonean mobilities in terms of care and as a response to a local health emergency. This framing also draws attention to the contradictory mobility dynamics that characterised British epidemic interventions in Freetown and West Africa more generally. The mobilisation of British expertise in the form of several medical officers stands in stark contrast to the quarantine imposed on Freetown according to the report. This foreshadows similar dynamics visible during the 2014–16

Ebola epidemic, in which lockdowns were imposed on the entire Sierra Leonean population (BBC, 2015) while international health responders travelled to and within Sierra Leone to work in the response. As in 1913, the 2014–16 Ebola epidemic was characterised by the simultaneous mobilisation of European-based expertise and immobilisation of Freetown under quarantine or quarantine-like measures.

The ships on which Rubert Boyce travelled from England to Sierra Leone and then on to Ghana were, in the years following the yellow fever outbreak, replaced by aeroplanes. White British mobility continued to be encouraged. As with the management of diseases, the British empire relied on mobilities between the different colonies and with the UK. The rapid propagation of air travel at the beginning of the twentieth century also extended to colonial Africa. Aeromobilities played an active role in making territories accessible for colonisation and developing them according to colonial doctrines. As Peter Adey (2010, p. 87) argued in relation to early aerial surveys: 'the aerial view revealed a reality that demanded improvement and development'. With the aeroplane, the British empire could be tied together as new flight routes were discussed and new geographical perspectives could be developed (Zook and Brunn, 2006). During a discussion on imperial air routes at the Royal Geographical Society in 1920, attended by Winston Churchill, the then Secretary of State for Colonies, it was stated that 'the importance to the empire of the development of aviation is obvious' (Prince of Wales et al., 1920, p. 264). Aeromobilities not only served to connect different ends of the empire, aerial mapping technologies also increased the epistemic and strategic advantage of the UK over the territories that constituted its empire.

In the increasing availability of commercial flights, colonial expansion and aeromobilities came together. This is illustrated by the cover of an Imperial Airways flight schedule from 1931. Imperial Airways, a precursor of the British Overseas Airways Cooperation (BOAC) and British Airways (Deal et al., 2018) offered flights connecting London to India and Egypt, Sudan and East and South Africa, as part of its 'Empire Service' as early as 1931 (Figure 10). On an Imperial Airways flight schedule from October 1931, the aerial view that Adey (2010) described is depicted graphically (Dawes, n.d.). The view is that of an aeroplane approaching Africa and India from the south. The empire in this image is laid out in front of the viewer – Africa below, Asia to the right – who can trace the airline's route from Cape Town to London and from Cairo to Delhi. Although the British colonial dream of a railway connection linking Cape Town to Cairo failed, aeromobilities achieved exactly that by opening up the empire commercially through speedy trans-imperial connections. For the white British traveller, the empire became a place of boundless mobility and circulation.

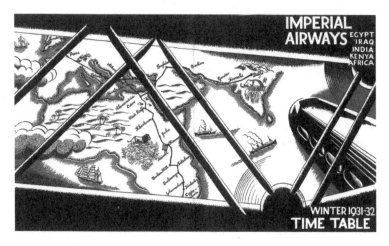

Figure 10   Imperial Airways October 1931 'Empire' routes. (Cover image from the collection of Michael Dawes, reprinted with permission)

West Africa was added to Imperial Airways' schedule in 1937 with connections to Nigeria and Ghana. From 1948, the West African Airways Cooperation (WAAC), jointly co-owned by British West African colonies, started offering flights to Freetown as part of its intercolonial service. To advertise these mobilities to the British public, WAAC advertisements were placed in targeted publications, such as *West Africa*, a weekly news magazine, published in London, highlighting West Africa's commercial and resource importance to the British empire and to Britain because of its geographical proximity. One such advertisement encouraged readers to 'Fly by the airmail routes' and promotes 'a comprehensive network of routes to 25 centres within West Africa' (TNA, CO1045/515). The WAAC encouraged white British civilians to explore West Africa through existing colonial air routes, contributing to the blurring of British colonisers and civilians. Through aeromobilities, British civilians could experience the empire in new and direct ways.

Freetown was linked through the WAAC to the capitals of other British West African colonies, such as Banjul, Accra and Lagos. In a 1951 article published in *Flight* magazine, a British journalist, Geoffrey Dorman (1951, pp. 38–40) describes this 'inter-colonial route' as having first been devised to facilitate the regional mobility of British colonial administrators and link West African colonies to Dakar and Khartoum. Although not explicitly racially segregated, the cost of an airline ticket prevented the vast majority of Black Sierra Leoneans from flying within West Africa, let alone from flying to the UK. In 1950 a second-class service was added to 'tap the African "man in the street" for their future potential' (Dorman, 1951, p. 39), illustrating that earlier routes had mostly been taken up by white European passengers. However, this service was not available on routes connecting Freetown to other cities. In 1951, a single fare from Freetown to London via Dakar cost £96, equivalent to over £2,000 today. The WAAC received technical advice from and acted as agent for BOAC (Dorman, 1951, pp. 38–40). West African aeromobilities were both devised and ensured by British expertise and colonial interests. They were largely organised around linking smaller colonies to West African colonial centres in Nigeria and Senegal. A direct route to London only operated to and from Dakar and Kano (northern Nigeria) (Dorman, 1951, p. 40). Starting in 1951, BOAC added Freetown to its world route. Through the aeroplane, access to and within Britain's colonies was facilitated. White mobility to and within West Africa was encouraged. Through mobility regulations, Blackness was construed as risky and deviant and independent Black mobility from Sierra Leone to the UK was actively discouraged.

In the case of Black Sierra Leoneans wanting to travel to London, mobility regulations applied to the 'native' population. Writing about a (white) Western conceptualisation of Blackness, Mbembe (2017, p. 28) argues that 'its function first and foremost [was] to codify the conditions for the appearance and the manifestation of a racial subject that would be called the Black Man and, later, within colonialism, the Native (L'indigène)'.[4] In colonialism, 'Blackness' and 'Nativeness' become akin in that both are antithetical to whiteness. In the shift from enslaved to colonial mobilities, the regulation of Black mobility is framed through the figure of the native. An advertisement in a 1911 Sierra Leone Royal Gazette (TNA, CO271/17, p. 55) reads as follows:

Warning
Natives of this Colony and Protectorate who may be desirous of proceeding to England in search of employment are warned of the impossibility of obtaining employment there, and the danger which they run of getting stranded in that country if they go without sufficient funds. They are further warned that they are likely to find themselves in trouble

unless they have work assured to them on their arrival, or have the means to take them back if they fail in their object.

9th of February, 1911

From the founding of the Sierra Leone Company 120 years earlier, the undesirability of a Black presence in London had been British governmental policy. With the rise of regular ship and flight connections Black mobilities towards the UK had to be actively discouraged to preserve the illusion of whiteness of British cities. It is made clear here that most 'native' mobilities towards the UK, and their subsequent presence in Britain, are undesired. Black or native mobility towards the UK is framed as risky and is criminalised. This stands in stark contrast to the aeromobilities which invited British civilians to 'fly by the airmail routes'. The warning also signals the containment of the 'circulation of underdeveloped and non-insured life' (Duffield, 2008, p. 143), a marker of the difference between 'developed' and 'underdeveloped' nations. In the case of Sierra Leonean–British mobilities, Blackness is produced as risky and its mobility as deviant.

Today, the directionality of mobilities is still unevenly immersed in postcolonial geographies and power dynamics. This became obvious during the Ebola epidemic, during which postcolonial visa and health regulations precluded the majority of mobilities from Sierra Leone to the UK. This impacted the capacity of Sierra Leonean and African healthcare workers to take part in the epidemic response. Anton explained the constraints that his organisation was subject to in recruiting healthcare workers to the Sierra Leonean response:

What would have helped would have been if they [the British government, WHO] confirmed that medevacs were gonna be available for any nationality and how that was gonna be sorted. That wasn't done. So we knew British people would get out, we knew someone from Spain would be alright, we didn't know if any of our Kiwi staff were. To be honest we were told pretty clearly if they were from the right type of Commonwealth country they'd be alright. Like that was the indication [...]. I think we did not take volunteers from other African countries because we didn't know what would happen if they got sick.

Anton's quote illustrates the entanglement of postcolonial mobility politics and the organisation of an epidemic response. His statement that medevacs (aerial evacuations to specialised hospitals) would not be made available to African healthcare workers or staff originating from 'the wrong type of Commonwealth country' was mirrored in newspaper articles (Harker, 2014; Benton, 2014) and in the reluctance to medevac Dr Khan or Dr Buck. His differentiation between 'the right type of Commonwealth country' and 'other African countries' indicates (post) colonial-racial hierarchies that underlay the response, but which for the most part were not openly addressed. Apart from the reproduction of colonial mobility dynamics themselves, these politics also led to a reification of both Sierra Leone and Africa more generally as unable to care for itself, as not possessing qualified healthcare workers and as having to rely heavily on the mobilisation of white European and North American volunteers to save Sierra Leonean lives.

Contrary to Sheppard's (2002) argument, the control over the directionality and nature of movements was and is important in the determination of aeromobilities. The control over mobilities shapes and was shaped by Britain's understanding of Sierra Leone as an extractive, non-settler colony. Economic interests played an important role in this control. The warning published in the Sierra Leone *Royal Gazette* seemed to be targeted largely against the 'threat' of homeless, jobless Africans in the streets of Britain, the very undesirability of which had contributed to the foundation of the colony of Sierra Leone (and their subsequent resettlement in Sierra Leone) (Fyfe, 1962; Olusoga, 2016).

Present aeromobilities, of course, are highly dependent on economic calculations as well. British Airways' decision to suspend the Freetown–London route during and after the Sierra Leonean Ebola epidemic was purportedly based on financial grounds. At the same time, Europe's current visa policies, which made the repatriation of non-European (non-white) healthcare workers so difficult, is also motivated by fears of foreign beneficiaries of the welfare state.[5] Migrants (and refugees) are still 'warned that they are likely to find themselves in trouble unless they have work assured to them on their arrival' (TNA, CO271/17, p. 55). The continuation of these dynamics signals the colonial wake. The directionality of mobilities is imbued with antiblackness and produces Blackness as deviant and risky.

Colonial Infrastructures

In *Zong!* (Philip and Boateng, 2011), M. NourbeSe Philip laments the massacre by the captain and crew of the *Zong*, a British slave ship from which

150 enslaved Africans were thrown overboard on its way to Jamaica in 1781. Due to navigational errors, the ship had run out of potable water and the crew drowned that number of enslaved Africans so as to be able to claim insurance on behalf of the ship's owners.[6] *Zong!* also laments the violence and meagreness of the legal language contained in *Gregson v. Gilbert*, the legal case report and only surviving written document attesting to the massacre. *Gregson v. Gilbert* is an insurance, not a murder case, and the language of the report attests to this:

> This was an action on a policy of insurance, to recover the value of certain slaves thrown overboard for want of water. The declaration stated, that by the perils of the seas, and contrary currents and other misfortunes, the ship was rendered foul and leaky, and was retarded in her voyage; and, by reason thereof, so much of the water on board the said ship, for her said voyage, was spent on board the said ship: that before her arrival at Jamaica, to wit, on, &c. a sufficient quantity of water did not remain on board the said ship for preserving the lives of the master and mariners belonging to the said ship, and of the negro slaves on board, for the residue of the said voyage; by reason whereof, during the said voyage, and before the arrival of the said ship at Jamaica – to wit, on, &c. and on divers days between that day and the arrival of the said ship at Jamaica – sixty negroes died for want of water for sustenance; and forty others, for want of water for sustenance, and through thirst and frenzy thereby occasioned, threw themselves into the sea and were drowned; and the master and mariners, for the preservation of their own lives, and the lives of the rest of the negroes, which for want of water they could not otherwise preserve, were obliged to throw overboard 150 other negroes. (*Gregson v. Gilbert 1783*, in Philip and Boateng, 2011, p. 210)

Philip disintegrates the language of *Gregson v. Gilbert* to 'not tell the story that must be told' (Philip and Boateng, 2011, p. 189). In 'Ferrum', *Zong!*'s penultimate chapter, she writes (2011, p. 138):

```
              on                              ce now she
   re               ad s rapt th        is story
        yarn a tale              which w
              ill not be              told yet w      ill have it
   s say it               is a wh            ore age w
```

In *Gregson v. Gilbert* what was at stake was the ship's distress and whether the latter was occasioned by navigational errors on behalf of the captain or 'perils of the seas' (Philip and Boateng, 2011, p. 211). It is impossible to debate *Gregson v. Gilbert* without reproducing the epistemic and physical violence which occasioned the trial in the first place. What ties the language of *Gregson v. Gilbert* to that of the colonial texts I discuss below is how the stripping of African humanity and agency is obscured by overly technical texts and a foregrounding of infrastructures, rather than the antiblackness they enable. Sharpe (2016, p. 37) speaks to this in her discussion of *Zong!*, even if only indirectly, when she draws attention to the distinction between the figure of the slave and that of the ship in contemporary accounts. Upon arrival in Jamaica a local newspaper commented on the ship's distress (navigational errors, prolonged journey) rather than that of the enslaved. Sharpe writes: 'Here, if not everywhere, as we will see, the ship is distinct from the slave.' In the case of the *Zong*, this distinction of personifying the ship yet denying the enslaved personhood is a further sign of antiblackness, A focus on the ship as distinct from the enslaved moves attention to the ship as an infrastructure on which the slave trade and colonialism relied. These infrastructures, the routes and materials they rely on, endure and can be analysed as continually producing Blackness as dependency. To see 'the ship [a]s distinct from the slave' allows a focus on ships and aeroplanes as constituting colonial and antiblack infrastructures after enslavement and colonialism. Infrastructures and aeromobilities in particular played an important role in the development of colonialism (Adey, 2010, p. 87). The economic and social development of colonial regions was seen as a central justification for investing in and building aeromobile infrastructures:

> The infrastructure of air-routes and pathways necessary to conduct aerial photography would have to be built, constructing a symbolic and material presence in colonial regions – the aerial survey as harbinger of development. Requiring considerable infrastructure to support the mobilities and maintenance of aircraft, air survey was a conduit through which development could be piped. The infrastructure necessary for air-routes and commercial services could already be in place for colony development. (Adey, 2010, p. 87)

In the wake, these infrastructures produce Sierra Leone and its population as dependent on British aid and expertise. In this section I focus on these enduring infrastructures and the colonial considerations that led to the building of and investment in material mobility infrastructures in Sierra Leone. Human infrastructures, or 'people as infrastructure' (Simone, 2004), were an instrumental part in British efforts to remain a central player in the development of West African aeromobilities post-independence. Both types of infrastructures played important roles during the 2014–16 Ebola epidemic and carry the colonial past into the present.

On the eve of independence the colonial government invested in aeromobile infrastructures in Sierra Leone. In 1960, it proposed the construction of a new, bigger airfield in Kenema, in eastern Sierra Leone, to be funded through a Colonial Development and Welfare fund.[7] The following excerpt is from internal communications between the British Treasury, the Colonial Office and the Communications Department regarding the construction of said airfield and the extension of Lungi airport:

> Mr Wallace also mentioned that Kenema was of importance from an internal security point of view since it was the nearest possible point to the diamond mining areas, and if trouble occurred there it might be necessary to organise an airlift of troops or police. In that event a runway of conventional length which would take fairly large sized aircraft was necessary. (TNA, CO937/510)

The 'trouble' anticipated in this communication imagines Blackness as an internal security threat, which can be controlled through aeromobilities. One year prior to independence, this security threat around diamond mining in eastern Sierra Leone was an important matter for the colonial government, which they sought to address through improved aeromobilities. The building of a new airstrip, which, in the internal communications was discussed in financial and temporal terms (the airstrip having to be financed from local funds from the day of independence on 21 April 1961), enabled (post)colonial aeromobile access to Sierra Leone's diamond-rich eastern region. Further to establishing a colonial presence in Sierra Leone, the infrastructures that supported colonial mobilities endure into the present. The Kenema airfield, for instance was used by the United Nations Humanitarian Air Service, a branch of the World Food Programme, during the Ebola response (Logistics Cluster, 2022). Aeromobile infrastructures were seen to grant police and military speedy access to and from Sierra Leonean diamond fields, which at the time were controlled by the British colonial government and London-based British-South African firm De Beers (Smilie et al., 2000) which operated a diamond field near Kenema. As with Kenema, infrastructure investments for Lungi airport's extension are discussed in British colonial communications. Lungi airport, situated across the estuary from Freetown is presently Sierra Leone's only international airport. It was converted from a pre-existing RAF (Royal Air Force) base into an airport in the 1950s by the British colonial government (TNA, CO937/262). Similar to Kenema airport, the airport's expansion by British colonial powers was linked to security concerns. In 1953, a communiqué between the Air Ministry and the Colonial Office revealed the following:

The War Office has asked us [Air Ministry] to prepare a plan for the reinforcement of Sierra Leone in the event of civil disturbances as part of Operation 'Weary' which covers the West African Colonies.[8] Unfortunately the only airfield of any size in Sierra Leone (Freetown/Lungi) has, according to our latest information, an all-up weight limitation of 50,000 lbs and hence appears to be unsuitable for Hastings, which would be operating at 70/75,000 lbs.[9] In all other respects however the airfield is acceptable, and Transport Command would be willing to operate Hastings from it in an emergency, provided the weight limitation could be temporarily raised. [...] If smaller aircraft had to be used, we should need to have more of them or to make more journeys, or both, and this would involve greater expense and possibly some delay in completing the operation. (TNA, CO937/262)

In both cases – the construction of Kenema and Lungi airfields – security concerns are written into material and financial calculations around aeroplane types and weight, landing-strip length and weight limitation. What is discussed here are the technological requirements to clamp down on political protest, framed as 'civil disturbances'. The reinforcement of Lungi and Kenema airfields was discussed to grant speedy access to parts of the empire that needed to be controlled and in which political and socio-economic uprisings needed to be quelled. The excerpt indicates one more point: until the late 1950s and until the political situation on the ground seemed to demand greater security, British colonial officers in Sierra Leone did not deem a bigger airport necessary. Existing infrastructure was sufficient to ensure colonial mobilities (always in relatively small numbers) throughout the region and on to London. Sierra Leonean aeromobilities were not designed for popular Sierra Leonean use.[10] This reinforces an image of Sierra Leone as a place of resource extraction, which was (and is) largely ensured by ships. Sierra Leonean mobilities were organised around a British understanding of Sierra Leone as a dependent place. This echoes the production of Blackness as dependence, which was used as a justification for British colonisation (Mbembe, 2001, 2017). In the conception of Sierra Leone's aeromobilities, Sierra Leoneans' mobilities were barely considered. Rather, the conception of colonial aeromobilities was designed to ensure the continued protection of British interests. A development of Simone's (2004) concept of 'people as infrastructure' illustrates this.

Writing about inner-city Johannesburg, Simone (2004) offers 'people as infrastructure' to think through the ever-moving, socially heterogeneous dynamics of urban Africa. He argues (2004, p. 411) that: 'people as infrastructure describes a tentative and often precarious process of remaking the inner city, especially now that the policies and economies that once moored it to the surrounding city have mostly worn away'.[11]

Here I want to extend Simone's (2004) concept to think through colonial mobility infrastructures in Sierra Leone. I propose that at the moment of independence the material infrastructures, put in place by Sierra Leone's colonial government, which would allow the future of aeromobilities into Sierra Leone, were supplemented by human expertise and skills in the form of seconded BOAC advisors and experts. This reliance on white 'people as infrastructure' reiterates the colonial-racial mobility injustice at the heart of British–Sierra Leonean relations. White expertise is mobilised to shape the future of Sierra Leonean mobilities according to British interests.

The independence of participating states in the late 1950s and early 1960s saw the end of the WAAC and the emergence of national carriers. A 1960 British government report on civil aviation in Sierra Leone, discussing future Sierra Leonean aeromobilities, focuses on how the impending independence of Nigeria led to fears of a disruption to flight services linking Sierra Leone to the rest of the region and to the UK (TNA, CO937/544). Colonial governance had ensured continued British aerial access financially, materially and politically in West Africa through the joint ownership of the WAAC by British West African colonies. At the moment of independence this access, and the economic advantages that it promised, were thrown into question. While the report states that it is politically 'impracticable for either the French or ourselves to make any direct attempt to re-assert our control over traffic rights in this area', it also encourages the possibility of 'avoiding the placing of unnecessary restriction on the freedom of our respective airlines' (TNA, CO937/544) in the development of West African aerial routes. Like the WAAC, the newly emerging national airlines, such as Sierra Leone Airways, Ghana Airways or Nigeria Airways, relied largely on expatriate BOAC workers and their skills in the establishment of their national carriers and the maintenance of existing equipment (TNA, CO937/544). UK representatives in Sierra Leone encouraged this involvement:

> The U.K. High Commissioner felt that it was very much in BOAC's interest to ensure that there was complete liaison between themselves as partners with the airlines in West Africa and BOAC (AC) Ltd. as shareholders in these airlines. The best men available should be nominated to serve with the West African associates. [...] there are also some grounds for believing that [West African] Ministers and officials are genuinely appreciative of the help so far received from BOAC even although they are chary of expressing such sentiments which would ill accord with the popular idea of independence. (TNA, CO937/544)

Aeromobilities and the future access of BOAC, which would later become British Airways, were negotiated at the moment of West African independence (1957–65) and the maintenance of close links was deemed important to fulfil British interests in West Africa. This was done to counteract the shift from WAAC, an airline designed to serve and rely on intercolonial routes and infrastructures, to national airlines in which British ownership and control was less direct. To maintain British influence and with regard to securing continued access to West African countries, 'the best men available should be nominated to serve with West African associates' (TNA, CO937/544).

For the material infrastructures in which the colonial government had invested to ensure British aeromobilities (in the form of British airlines such as BOAC), British negotiators built on human expertise and skill. The shift from outright British government control to BOAC shareholdership necessitated the skilled negotiation techniques of BOAC representatives in coordination with UK government representation on the ground. To be able to convince newly independent states that existing aeromobile infrastructures should guarantee continued British access, the political atmosphere had to be carefully read and negotiated with delicacy (TNA, CO937/544):

the position of BOAC nominated directors and of skilled managerial and technical staff seconded by BOAC is extremely difficult. It is often apparent to them that government intervention or support will be necessary to secure the adoption of sound policies or the correction of abuses but if they approach Ministers or officials they are vulnerable to the charges that they are going over the heads of the board or that they are intriguing behind the backs of government appointed directors. Occasionally this risk can be avoided by arranging for the approach to government to be made by a visiting representative of BOAC, not holding office in the local airline, where BOAC can allege a legitimate interest in the matter at issue because of its bearing on the prospects of the partnership between BOAC and the national airline [...].

This passage shows the importance of human infrastructure in the bid for continued British aeromobilities throughout West Africa. The material infrastructures put in place in the 1950s, such as the building of Kenema and the extension of Lungi airfield, depended on skilled negotiators and political ruses to continue to be useful for British aviation. British interests rested on material *and* human infrastructures. The fears that Britain was to be excluded from West African aeromobilities here led to deception and strategising, both of which relied on Britain's vast network of governmental and commercial representatives. In Sierra Leone, colonial future-making depended on material as well as human infrastructures. This becomes relevant in a reading of the 2014–16 British-led Ebola response, which mobilised a similar network of material and human infrastructure and in which (im)mobilities were similarly entangled with racist differentiation.

At Lungi airport, built under British colonial rule, baggage handling and security have since 2012 been managed by Westminster Group PLC, a British private security firm with a mandate to combat crime and increase efficiency (Bangura, 2015).[12] In a 2019 interview, their chairman Sir Tony Baldry stated that: 'We started operating in Sierra Leone in 2012 when the country was in dire need of a professional company to handle the ground handling of the Lungi airport. At that time we sent in 30 experts to work with Sierra Leoneans' (Thomas, 2019b). Through these material and human infrastructures – the 'experts' that Tony Baldry speaks of – the engineered dependency which characterises colonialism is extended. In the wake the management of Freetown International Airport depends on British experts travelling to and from Sierra Leone to regulate and enable mobilities in and out of the country. Before and after independence, Sierra Leonean aeromobilities are ensured through British governmental and private interests taking the form of material and human infrastructures. Here, colonial continuities and concurrences work their way through the wake.

In the case of Sierra Leone, Blackness has long been produced through the framing and regulation of colonial mobilities. Routes, directionality and infrastructures are just three entry points into an exploration of how mobilities constitute the colonial wake and contributed to shifting definitions of Blackness. Rather than demonstrating explicit causality, I have tried to present a picture of the sweeping intersection of mobilities, antiblackness and British colonialism in Sierra Leone. As in the previous chapter, the colonial wake here does not take exclusively material form. Aeromobilities relied and continue to rely on colonial infrastructures, which in Sierra Leone take both material and human form.

The preceding is a necessary backdrop for an analysis of British–Sierra Leonean mobilities during the 2014–16 Ebola response; for an analysis that knows the wake. While I explore contemporary mobilities, I draw attention to the political and geographical concurrences and disruptions whose colonial basis I have mapped out here. As per Stoler's (2016, p. 117) invitation to think about a colony as 'a principle of managed migration' I examine UK–Sierra Leonean colonial relations through an analysis of the politics of mobility. In the next section I suggest that mobilities during and after the Ebola epidemic continue to shape Blackness as dependency and were themselves perceived as multiple. These multiple mobilities create multiple Sierra Leones, on which in turn a contemporary Black diasporic ontology depends.

Contemporary Mobilities and Mobile Ontologies

In this section I attend to contemporary mobilities and the multiple mobile ontologies they create. I argue that the suspension of direct flights between London and Freetown, and reactions to it, recall the careful production of Black Sierra Leoneans and Sierra Leone itself as dependent on the UK and on white expertise. Here, mobilities, their flow and interruption, their regulation and experience, signal the precarious postcolonial condition that shapes Black being and Sierra Leone in the wake.

Mbembe (2001, p. 13) argues that: 'the slave trade and colonialism echoed one another with the lingering doubt of the very possibility of self-government, and with the risk, which has never disappeared, of the continent and Africans being again consigned for a long time to a degrading condition'.

Following Mbembe (2001), I show that an analysis of the changing aeromobilities linking Sierra Leone and the UK during and after the Ebola epidemic reveals a continuing dependence and 'lingering doubt of the very possibility of self-government'. In the wake, Sierra Leonean mobilities still depend on white British expertise and material infrastructures. Black Sierra Leonean diasporic lives both depend on and invoke these (post)colonial flows and use them to subvert the construction of Sierra Leone as a place dependent on the UK. This signals the ongoing injustice at the heart of Sierra Leonean mobilities. As per Sheller's (2018, p. 21) definition of mobility injustice, I close this chapter by attending to the 'differential subjects', which the unequal, colonial and antiblack mobilities I have described here have created.

Aeromobilities in the Colonial Wake

The direct flight between London and Freetown has long been a focal point in Sierra Leonean–British aeromobilities. In post-civil war Sierra Leone only Brussels Airways' direct Freetown–Brussels international connection preceded BA's Freetown–London route, the former starting in 2002 and the latter in 2008. The British Airways route connecting Freetown to London was launched by bmi (British Midlands International) in 2008 and taken over by British Airlines after the airlines' merger in 2012 (Maslen, 2012). Gambia Bird, a subsidiary of German airline Germania, launched services in 2012 linking Freetown to London and to other regional capitals. Other routes gradually joined in the 2010s. During the Ebola epidemic however, all airlines except Brussels Airways and Royal Air Maroc suspended flights to Sierra Leone. While most airlines resumed their flights after the outbreak, British Airways CEO Alex Cruz declared the routes to be not 'commercially viable' in 2016 (Massaquoi, 2018).

The direct flights between the UK and Sierra Leone were an important part of diasporic lives. David, a member of the Sierra Leonean diaspora in the UK, described the importance of the direct connection and the lengths to which he went to have direct flights connecting London and Freetown reinstated. He also described how the suspension affected the diaspora in the UK:

Actually the suspension, interesting case, because I remember working on an advocacy effort to ask the UK government to lift the ban because the ban, we assumed that it was imposed by the UK government even though they denied it, and so I remember getting back a response from the Minister of Transport writing me back that the ban has actually been lifted. But then it was lifted in theory, but in practice there was still no direct route between the two because BA, which was flying directly, stopped during Ebola citing health issues, but then once the ban was lifted they never went back and that had some impact and that was the motivation for me to start the advocacy drive in the first place because a lot of Sierra Leoneans that I talked to especially those that had business interests in Sierra Leone, and also those that wanted to help out from a humanitarian point of view, didn't have an opportunity to fly from here to Sierra Leone and instead they had to go to a different country and some weren't even able to make it. So, it deprived the response as well from a humanitarian angle not just from a business perspective.

David's account signals the diaspora's quotidian reliance on direct flights, but also their desire to be involved in the Ebola response. His statement that 'some weren't even able to make it' indicates a feeling of dependence, which weaves its way through this chapter and which is echoed by other members of the diaspora further down. Furthermore, the direct route was perceived by some Sierra Leoneans in Sierra Leone and in the diaspora as an appreciation of Sierra Leone by the former colonial power.

Upon the inauguration of Gambia Bird's Freetown–London route a Sierra Leonean journalist reported the following: 'While urging the airline to ensure that they give the British Airways a run for their money with their new route to London via Freetown, Minister Koroma [Minister for Transport and Aviation] pointed out that London is a preferred route for Sierra Leoneans because of the rich colonial ties between the two countries' (Tarawallie, n.d.). These rich colonial ties were often invoked by members of the Sierra Leonean diaspora too. Two online petitions, one on *change.org* the other on *38degrees.com* urged British Airways, not Gambia Bird, to resume direct flights to Sierra Leone. The texts of both petitions made explicit links to Sierra Leone's colonial past. Tony Rogers, a British healthcare worker who was part of the British response to Sierra Leone launched the *38degrees* petition in 2015. In his petition he quotes an editorial from Sierra Leonean newspaper *Torchlight* (Rogers, 2015):

Sierra Leoneans felt abandoned by the former colonial masters when even an attempt by Gambia Bird Airlines to resume direct flights was met with stiff rejection from the British government.

Similarly, Martha Massaquoi, who set up the *change.org* petition in 2016, stated that:

As a Commonwealth country, we feel that the link to the UK provided by British Airways represented an important bond between the countries. (Massaquoi, 2016)

Britain's colonial history in Sierra Leone was also taken up by some of the signatories who commented on the *change.org* petition (see Massaquoi, 2016, 2018). Out of 701 signatories, 266 people commented, some only writing their names, some writing lengthy explanations as to why they wanted BA to resume flights (Massaquoi, 2018). A 'direct' route or flights were mentioned 81 times, making it the prime reason why people signed. Allusions to Britain's colonial past in Sierra Leone took different forms. A direct route between Britain and Sierra Leone was seen as a sign of a privileged relationship due to the countries' shared colonial past. At the same time this reflects the careful construction of both Blackness and Sierra Leone as a colony, that is, as a place/race whose autonomy is perpetually in doubt (Mbembe, 2001, 2017). Some comments made direct reference to colonialism, while others wrote about the commonwealth or shared history:

Sierra Leone was British Colonized until our independence in 1961. In light of that, Britain should be more sympathetic to Sierra Leoneans especially in time of devastation (EBOLA, MUDSLIDE etc.). I am doubtful as far as their loyalty to Sierra Leone when our people are abandoned during their time of crises by a country that colonized them for so long. They stopped all flights to Sierra Leone, it was only SN Brussels that stuck with us during these difficult times and I commend them for their patriotism. [...] (Seray Dumbuya, in Massaquoi, 2018)

Because Sierra Leone is a former British colonial country. And families are suffering to travel to Freetown or London. (Mohamed Amara Samba Mustapha, in Massaquoi, 2016)

Direct flights to Sierra Leone is a necessity. Britain needs to stand by Sierra Leone. (Rebecca Yongawo, in Massaquoi, 2016)

Ebola is now finished and all their fears have proved wrong. Royal Air Maroc & SN Brussels flew through out [sic] the whole episode and no lives were put at risk. In addition we have a long history with BA and UK as Sierra Leone is an old British Colony. (Frances Fode, in Massaquoi, 2016)

I wholeheartedly support this long overdue request for a vital service that is not only financially beneficial to the countries but also cements the historical bond between our countries and peoples. (Saeley Johnson, in Massaquoi, 2016)

I believe it benefits the company, the two states and above all it cements the ties between us as a commonwealth country. (Patrick Lebbie, in Massaquoi, 2016)

There is a huge diaspora of Sierra Leoneans in the UK and a long history of links between the countries. [...] Direct air travel between the UK and this commonwealth country is essential. (Douglas Laurie, in Massaquoi, 2016)

In these comments, current direct aeromobilities are seen as 'cementing' historical ties and bonds between the two countries. Furthermore, the former colonial relation between Sierra Leone and the UK is expressed emotionally. 'Britain needs to stand by Sierra Leone', 'I am doubtful as far as their loyalty' or 'their fears have proved wrong' all indicate that for the people commenting on the petition, BA's decision to suspend flights during the Ebola epidemic and to extend the suspension affected them emotionally. These emotions signal the colonial present; a present in which the colonial past translates into a privileged special relationship between Britain and its former colonies. Here the colonial and antiblack violence that has characterised Britain's role in Sierra Leone for so long is relegated or invoked to form an emotional bond that would lead BA to reinstate a flight connection, which for them was no longer profitable (Massaquoi, 2018). The comments indicate a sense that Britain 'owed' Sierra Leone, or that it should 'care' about Sierra Leone and the ways in which this suspension affected Sierra Leonean lives in the diaspora and at home. This sense was confirmed by Brima, a member of the Sierra Leonean community in the UK. When speaking to me about the flights he said:

British Airways [...] have still not resumed flights to Sierra Leone which to me is kind of a lesson to us Sierra Leoneans. I think we tend to think the British care about us; they don't even know we exist until something like Ebola happens.

For Brima, the suspension of direct flights was revealing of British attitudes towards Sierra Leone. Taken in conjunction with Minister Koroma's statement, which framed Sierra Leonean–British aeromobilities as an expression of 'rich colonial ties', Brima's statement suggests that in the case of Sierra Leonean–British aeromobilities, a direct connection was seen by many Sierra Leoneans as a British appreciation of Sierra Leone, whereas a suspension of the direct route was seen as a lack of care and loyalty. By contrast, no online petitions were directed towards Gambia Bird to resume flights connecting London and Freetown. Brima's statement also makes clear that, for him, the Ebola epidemic had revealed the extent to which these feelings were one-sided and belonged to the past. The British had reduced Sierra Leone and the mobilities which tied it to the UK to the Ebola epidemic and the threat the virus posed to the UK population. Mobilities were reconfigured to fit the Ebola aftermath, one in which the threat of infection had subsided, but in which pre-Ebola conditions were not reinstated. Ebola had thus made it harder for Sierra Leoneans in the diaspora to travel to Freetown, not only because of the virus, but because of a new postcolonial power geography in which Sierra Leonean–British mobilities had been further marginalised. 'The British', in other words, did not care about 'rich colonial ties' or the long-standing mobilities between London and Freetown. In the wake of colonialism and Ebola, Black mobilities between the two countries were once again made more difficult and the contribution and exploitation of Black life in creating these very mobilities in the first place were marginalised. At the same time, Brima's disillusionment reflects his inability, and that of the diaspora, to hold sway over places increasingly drawn together through airlines and those left aside.

Multiple Mobile Ontologies

Disruptions experienced by members of the Sierra Leonean diaspora in the UK in comparison to narrations by international health responders indicate Sierra Leone's multiple 'mobile ontologies' (Sheller, 2018). As a reminder, Sheller (2018, p. 9) defines mobile ontologies as ontologies 'in which *movement is primary as a foundational condition of being, space, subjects, and power* [...]'. The ways in which mobilities between the two countries, their flows and disruptions, were understood by interviewees show Sierra Leone's multiple mobile ontologies. Whereas the (predominantly white) international health responders I interviewed described the disruption through its effects on the organisation of the response and consequently construed Sierra Leone as a place in need of foreign intervention, members of the diaspora (entirely Black) construed the country as a place of economic opportunity.[13] This last point is especially indicative of a Black diasporic mobile ontology which infers British–Sierra Leonean mobilities that differ from the mobilities of extraction and intervention that characterised the colonial period and the Ebola epidemic. Whereas throughout this chapter I have pointed to the production of Blackness as ontological negation, deviance and dependence, here I point to Black African sovereign mobilities, which occur in the wake, but subvert historical dynamics.

The diaspora experienced the suspension of flights differently from international responders, many of whom did not comment on it at all because it did not affect them beyond the extraordinary moment of this particular Ebola response. (This is the impermanent nature of humanitarian action – it constructs places in the short-term.) For the diaspora, the suspension of flights was concerning for reasons that went beyond Ebola and the humanitarian emergency that unfolded in Sierra Leone. This is not to say that they were indifferent to Ebola, rather, at the time of our interviews, the threat of Ebola had passed and the reality of there being no direct air route between Freetown and London, with all its economic and social implications, was still present. From their perspective, suspending the flights disrupted quotidian mobilities that connected their lives in the UK and Sierra Leone. Despite the availability of new (indirect) routes connecting London and Freetown, and Freetown to the world, offered by a variety of regional and international airlines in the aftermath of the Ebola epidemic, members of the Sierra Leonean diaspora focused on the lack of direct flights. Direct flights represented an opportunity to live mobile lives and to conduct business in an environment in which their Sierra Leonean–British identities conferred a higher status than they did in the UK. These self-initiated mobilities are an important aspect of the Black diasporic experience and identity. Anxieties around the flights' suspension were articulated in terms of a loss of business opportunities. Among the members of the Sierra Leonean diaspora in the UK (and Europe) I interviewed, more than three quarters had been to Sierra Leone in the last five years or had immediate plans for visiting. Some, such as Aminata, owned businesses which operated entirely in Sierra Leone. Aminata's identity as a successful Sierra Leonean-British woman entrepreneur depended on her social enterprise, which in turn depended on speedy flight connections linking her life in London, where she moved with her parents during the civil war, and her desire to uplift marginalised women in Sierra Leone.

It was so easy for me because when I am taking my products, like when we done the pilot I just filled up all my suitcases instead of shipping, which I know I wouldn't have gotten it on time. And the BA was so good for me, straight direct flight, straight into Lungi [Freetown's Airport], cross over, easy. So that was out, even up to now BA is not flying there, I don't know, so we currently don't even have direct flights going into Sierra Leone. And that affects loads of businesses. Because when BA was flying, people were going in and out, making deals, staying a couple of days, coming back. That was about six and a half hours and you're there. So that affected the kind of infrastructure to do business in Sierra Leone.

Her opinion was echoed by David, but also by people signing the online petition to reinstate flights. Living between Sierra Leone and the UK was an integral part of Aminata's life and that of other members of the diaspora. 'Business' was mentioned numerous times in the reasons people gave on the petition to want a direct flight connection reinstated.

I'm signing this petition, because BA is missing a great economic opportunity in West Africa. The UK is Sierra Leone's most important market, and Sierra Leone is full of opportunity for UK businesses, especially in travel and tourism. (Benjamin Carey, in Massaquoi, 2016)

I travel to Freetown and Monrovia for business and with a direct flight would make this journey more frequently, increasing business for my firm and for Sierra Leone. (Victor Benjamin, in Massaquoi, 2016)

I am signing because I love my country and I want British Airways to continue running and it's good for business investment for Mama Salone [colloquial name for Sierra Leone]. (Abu Fofanah, in Massaquoi, 2016)

Similarly, 'family' and 'home' were mentioned numerous times as well:

> I am signing because I want the flight to be going to Sierra Leone please as I will be very grateful to be visiting my family thank you. (Katie Dauda, in Massaquoi, 2016)
>
> It makes my family life easier and safer to travel back home. (Ahmad Allie, in Massaquoi, 2016)
>
> I'm signing because it is difficult for a Sierra Leonean to get a direct flight back home from United Kingdom. And this has resulted in few people to travel back home. (Osman Vandi, in Massaquoi, 2016)

On the other hand, on the rare occasions that they spoke about the suspension, British-based health responders, who were predominantly white, saw the interruption in terms of its effects on the Ebola response. They too were opposed to it, but on medical grounds. In contrast to members of the Sierra Leonean diaspora their narrations construct mobilities towards Sierra Leone not as quotidian but as emergency mobilities. Tom, a British doctor working in Freetown stated that:

> BA still isn't flying direct, Gambia Bird shut down as a result, especially the early days you know Royal Air Maroc and Brussels [Airways], good on them, if we'd waited for the UN response to be doing all the transport, then, the country would have collapsed.

Gareth, a doctor who worked for the same organisation as Tom, confirmed this sense:

> So there wasn't much option in terms of flights. So I flew with whoever was flying on the day I needed to fly. I went from Heathrow and I went via, I think I went via Brussels. Although I didn't disembark. The flight was quite interesting because it wasn't a commercial flight. It was a – well it was a commercial flight but it wasn't a typical commercial flight insofar as that everyone on the flight was going there for a specific reason so it had a very different feel to it from a normal commercial flight.

Anton, an NGO worker, explained the decision to suspend flights as one motivated by public perception:

The British government I think got a call from the *Daily Mail* I think at some point querying 'why are there still direct flights?' So they stopped them. Immediately. [...] And what we understood at the time is that the health leadership in the UK was strongly pushing to allow direct flights and actually said it would be safer to only have direct flights between the two countries, because then you can monitor who is coming in and out. If everyone is having to change through Brussels or through Casablanca then you have people going all over Europe, and people mixing [in] all kinds of airports everywhere, whereas if you got direct flights you know what you're doing, but the optics of having direct flights, people coming, people being one flight away from the UK was too great for the government to risk going with.

Anton's quote indicates that the suspension was perceived as being motivated by British public opinion. His explanation that the health leadership in the UK sought to maintain direct flights is significant. Whether this is true or not, it is a further sign of the dependence of Sierra Leonean aeromobilities on UK public and private interests. Tom's emphasis that without Royal Air Maroc and Brussels Airways 'the country would have collapsed' shows the health emergency framing through which he perceived Sierra Leone, whose salvation was, once again, dependent on mobilities of British care. Likewise, Gareth's statement construes the aeromobilities connecting London and Freetown that he experienced as not 'normal'. Their narrations indicate that their mobile relations to Sierra Leone were temporary and based on the idea of Sierra Leone as a place in need of intervention. This temporariness is reminiscent of white colonial mobilities into Sierra Leone, which, unlike in settler colonies such as Australia or South Africa, were always temporary. In contrast to the diaspora's narrations their mobilities were not quotidian, but emergency mobilities.

The lives of members of the Sierra Leonean diaspora in the UK seemed to be more dependent on mobilities connecting the two countries than those of international health responders. Their relation to Sierra Leone is a long-standing one, whereas for the most part international responders' engagement was temporary. These differences contribute to Sierra Leone's multiple mobile ontologies. Here mobilities into and out of Sierra Leone have construed Sierra Leone as multiple places: as a place of economic opportunity or one in urgent need of foreign intervention on the brink of collapse. The mobilities of the diaspora differ from those of international health workers. Their mobilities construe Sierra Leone as a place of opportunity and as a place which has always existed in close relationship with the UK. For them the disruption of direct flights was perceived as a disruption of this long-standing relationship. For international health responders, on the other hand, Sierra Leone was a temporary place of crisis in need of temporary intervention. Here the mobilities that connect Sierra Leone and the UK and the place they create are multiple.

As during colonial times, the mobility and immobility, the flow and its disruption that connects and characterises British–Sierra Leonean relations is implicitly racial. In the long term, members of the Sierra Leonean diaspora suffered more from the disruption of direct flights than international health responders, for whom the initially temporary suspension did not have long-lasting effects. In the aftermath of the Ebola epidemic British Airways interrupted a flight connection that members of the diaspora (and the Sierra Leonean Minister for Transport and Aviation) perceived as an appreciation of Sierra Leonean–British relations and a shared past. It also constituted a crucial component of Black diasporic lives and signals a contemporary Black mobile ontology still characterised by mobility dependency while Black people are also living mobile lives that counteract the colonial wake. Calls for reinstating the flights were subsequently addressed to the British government and British Airways, signalling the persistent role that British actors and infrastructures play in ensuring Sierra Leonean aeromobilities. In the wake, and mirroring colonial and imperial dynamics, Sierra Leonean communities still depend on British private and governmental entities for their movement. Though nominally independent, Sierra Leone's mobilities towards the UK are a representation of postcolonial mobility injustice and the colonial-racial hierarchies that it entails.

Conclusion

The mobilities that have shaped Sierra Leone historically, during and in the aftermath of the 2014–16 Ebola epidemic are representative of and linked to the shifting production of (anti-)Blackness, described by Mbembe (2017) as 'Western consciousness of Blackness'. By tracing these shifting meanings through the mobilities and infrastructures that have linked Sierra Leone and the UK, I have sought to build on the importance that Black Studies has long placed on the transatlantic. In reproducing racial-colonial hierarchies Sierra Leonean–British mobilities are constitutive of the colonial wake. The establishment of routes, control over the directionality of flows and investment in colonial infrastructures have been entangled with the production of Blackness as ontological negation, deviance and dependence. Whereas British colonialism encouraged white quotidian mobilities between the UK and Sierra Leone, Black post-Ebola mobilities are increasingly made difficult and framed as exceptional. Sierra Leone's resulting mobile ontologies (Sheller, 2018) are multiple, and the mobilities are largely still dependent on the UK. Mobilities linking the two countries have been violent extractions of Black life and framed as mobilities of care; they have construed Sierra Leone as on the brink of collapse and in dire need of foreign aid but also as a place of economic opportunity.

The British-led Ebola response took place amidst – and exacerbated – the mobility injustice at the very centre of Sierra Leonean–British mobilities. Public health regulations and aeromobile infrastructures led to a situation in which Black Sierra Leonean immobility was set in opposition to white European and North American mobilisation towards Sierra Leone. At the same time I also see this analysis as a starting point to think through the inherent mobility of Black life. The case of Sierra Leone shows the extent to which mobilities linking Britain as imperial centre with its colonies were instruments of racial differentiation and laid the basis for a modern postcolonial mobility regime in which Black African mobility towards the UK (and Europe) is largely criminalised. At the same time, analysing the mobilities of members of Sierra Leonean diaspora in the UK has shown that a Black mobile ontology is also positive and self-initiated, and that it constitutes and depends on Sierra Leone as a place of economic opportunity. This echoes Sharpe's (2016, p. 16) recurring adage that:

> To be in the wake is also to recognize the ways that we are constituted through and by continued vulnerability to overwhelming force though not only known to ourselves and to each other by that force.

The contradictions at the heart of this Black mobile ontology, are deserving of future attention. In a post-Ebola world, Sierra Leone as a place of economic opportunity has been further relegated to the margins of British interest. The mobilities linking Sierra Leone to the UK have been further marginalised too, shaping and changing the lives of UK's Sierra Leonean diaspora. As during British colonialism, Sierra Leone's mobilities reify it as a place of underdevelopment and in need of (British) philanthropic care, underpinning its intended (post)colonial relationship of dependency.

3

Thinking and Practising Care: Space, Risk and Racialisation in Ebola Treatment Centres

Introduction

I do remember Bill taking a photo of a baby that had survived in Connaught's unit and showing me and giving me a photo and going: 'You did this because you got her out [of the community].' And that face made it all so much more worth it. Like, it just made me go 'Ok I can get up every day and I can do this.' At the same time had I met some more of those people I think then the problem was that actually I wouldn't have been able to do what I did and go home every night because then I would have started seeing faces to each of those names and at some point, I had to stop. So, I can sometimes understand why when you're in mass public emergency some people just – [pauses] – some people just have to deal with the names and switch off because if they had names and faces – like I would have internally imploded and actually probably just never stopped and you can't do that. You almost, almost start protecting yourself in there. It's like I can't see the people I don't want to see the people. [...]

I remember one day and this is the first day it happened and I was like 'This is a watershed moment and really really awful. This is how awful it is': I phoned up the unit, desperate for beds. Fatima went to me: 'Two people died overnight.' And I went: 'good' [laughs shortly]. And I went: 'Great'. And I stopped myself and I went 'Fuck', but it was the only way I could have coped was to – every woman every child every man, they were all the same.

And at that moment the only way to 'keep things moving' was if people died?

Yeah

Because that opened up new beds?

Yeah 'cause there were obstructions in testing so sometimes there were testing delays for three days [...] You think it was bad for me and then I think, you know and then you think there were people in those units for three fucking days four fucking days in these horrific units where they were shitting in fucking buckets. I can't even begin to think what that was like, but from my perspective it was like: I can't move anyone. And that was what was so weird. There'd be like massive productivity and then there'd be hours in the day when I was like [pauses]: There is nothing I can do right now. Nothing until someone dies or someone moves. Until one ambulance picks up, like manages to get that person to the treatment centre. They've picked them up and they call me and I say: 'Ok, this one person.' Ugh. (Anika, interview with the author, August 2017)

In this chapter I want to think through and with care. Doing so means attending to care practice in the context of the international Ebola response. Practice is an inherent part of medical care and here I focus on care practice as the individual exercise of medicine which, depending on practitioners, reflects a differential understanding of medicine's political or apolitical nature. However, I also want to think through these practices *with* care. By extending and challenging how we think of care and care practice and by borrowing and learning from epistemic communities that have thought care beyond its institutional boundaries. Such a focus on care, its various manifestations and conceptualisations, extends the historical entanglements between care and antiblack (and other forms of) violence which I have analysed in chapter 1 and introduces novel understandings of what it might mean to care for Black life in an EVD epidemic. In this chapter I try to keep those deeply empathic ways of caring in mind as I go about an analysis of EVD care during the 2014–16 Sierra Leonean pandemic.

I abstain here from offering a distinct definition of *care*, acknowledging that care – analytical, political, physical, mental – takes many forms. But I want to offer some parameters to think *carefully*, so to speak; to re/imagine care beyond its institutional boundaries, which have invariably been used to contain, constrain and control Black and Brown life and the lives of those who did not fit our ableist, heteronormative mould. At the beginning of their (2016, p. 38) book *Care Work: Dreaming Disability Justice*, disability justice activist Leah Lakshmi Piepzna-Samarasinha offers a history of care in the context of the Americas:

With the arrival of white settler colonialism, things changed, and not in a good way. For many sick and disabled Black, Indigenous and brown people under transatlantic enslavement, colonial invasion, and forced labor, there was no such thing as state-funded care. Instead, if we were too sick or disabled to work, we were often killed, sold, or left to die, because we were not making factory or plantation owners money. Sick, disabled, Mad, Deaf, and neurodivergent people's care and treatment varied according to our race, class, gender, and location, but for the most part, at best, we were able to evade capture and find ways of caring for ourselves or being cared for by our families, nations, or communities – from our Black and brown communities to disabled communities. At worst, a combination of legal and societal ableism plus racism and colonialism meant that we were locked up in institutions or hospitals, 'for our own good.'

Care took many of the same forms on the other side of the Atlantic under European colonialisms. As I continue to argue, the geographical divide between antiblack experiences of enslavement and antiblack experiences of colonialism speaks to differential manifestations of white supremacy globally. Thus, in this chapter I undertake a dual analysis of care as both institutional (and at times violent and antiblack) and care as that which exceeds and counteracts such instances of violence and exclusion. I want to put forward here, that in the case of the Sierra Leonean EVD epidemic, pushing the analytical and political boundaries of how we think about care and care practice also involves rethinking the parameters of what it means to be human. Care here constitutes an acknowledgement of the colonial parameters that have shaped how we see, understand and approach the human both in its conceptual and physical form.

During the epidemic care was shaped by three central factors. First, the absence of an Ebola cure. At the beginning of the West African Ebola outbreak in December 2013, no certified medicine or vaccine slowing or hindering the progress of EVD in the human body had been approved by the US Food and Drug Administration or similar national bodies. Second, the highly infectious nature of the disease and, third, the emergency setting, which required a makeshift approach to care materials and spaces. This chapter explores how these three factors shaped the caring practices available to and required by (clinical and non-clinical) international medical responders during the Ebola epidemic. That is, how international responders practised care in such an environment and how they conceived of and navigated the risks involved in their care work. In line with my central argument, I write to make the antiblackness which has shaped this epidemic response and others visible in responders' care practices.

While I draw on ontopolitics as a methodology and as an analytical concept, there are some marked differences between Annemarie Mol's (2002) analysis and mine. For one, Ebola is an infectious disease, not a chronic condition (like atherosclerosis, which Mol studies) and, as I will show, this has consequences for how its ontologies are enacted. Second, I explore how the ontologies of Ebola are enacted entirely within the international Ebola response to Sierra Leone, which constitutes an '(extra)ordinary event', in comparison to the everyday hospital setting in which Mol (2002) studies the ontopolitics of atherosclerosis.[1] Third, while my focus lies on practices of care, the nature of my research means that I explore these practices through the narrations of interviewees, not through participant observation, which forms the basis of Mol's (2002) work. Last, and relatedly, Mol (2002) makes a distinct differentiation between perspectives and realities. According to her (2002, pp. 10–13), perspectives, which are inherently personal, do not grasp the multiplicity of ontologies, but '"merely" interpret them'. I challenge this statement and its implicit hierarchy. Historical instances of antiblack violence (the slave trade, colonialism) shape embodied perspectives along racial-colonial lines to different degrees and those perspectives, in turn, shape the ontologies of the wake. Mol (2002, p. 55) raises the importance of geographical context by stating that 'ontology in medical practice is bound to a specific site and situation'. However, her analysis does not take the political history of such sites into account. This chapter speaks to my grappling with Mol's (2002) method: my approach adopts an ontopolitical stance in the study of medical practice, while also centring perspectives. This centring of perspectives is important, because who practises care, and where, matters, given the colonial-racial legacies of health and disease management in Sierra Leone and globally.

Practising Care, Thinking the Wake, Rethinking the Human

Thinking Care and Violence

Historical uses of care as violence are a marker of the wake and awareness of care's historical uses is a practice of care. When writing about thinking and practising care in the midst of the EVD epidemic, I want to extend this care to my analysis. This is an intellectual and methodological choice, inspired by the humanities, more than the social sciences perhaps. Black Studies has, for a long time, sought to do exactly that: to counter the violence Black people encounter with analyses that oppose simplistic rationalisations and narratives which perpetuate said violence. In her book *Wayward Lives, Beautiful Experiments*, Saidiya Hartman (2020, p. 31) describes her intellectual labour of recovering anonymous Black figures from archives and records: 'It was my way of redressing the violence of history, crafting a love letter to all those who had been harmed, and, without my being fully aware of it, reckoning with the inevitable disappearance that awaited me.'

Whereas the preceding chapters in this book have grappled with archival materials, this chapter is more anchored in the recent past and relies on interviews, discussions and observations. These constitute an archive of their own, one that grapples with care practices and caring for Black African lives in the wake of colonialism and, in the case of Sierra Leone, the civil war. Like Hartman, Sharpe also centres care and caring for Black life in her work. She writes:

> I want to think 'care' as a problem for thought. I want to think care in the wake as a problem for thinking and of and for Black non/being in the world. Put another way 'In the Wake: On Blackness and Being' is a work that insists and performs that thinking needs care and that thinking and care need to stay in the wake. (Sharpe, 2016, p. 5)

Similarly, here I want to think care into the EVD epidemic. This contributes to my overall aim of placing the Ebola response in the wake. Sharpe identifies care's multiple uses. In her own work, care is a methodology that structures her writing and analysis of the literary and visual representations she attends to. In her analysis of Black life in the wake, care is a shifting analytical field that encompasses both violence and the sharing of risk, a theme I return to in the second part of this chapter.

The historical and contemporary conflation between (biomedical) care and violence is one of the realities of living in the wake. However, in the interviews with international health responders I analyse here, antiblackness remains largely unheeded. In this section and throughout this chapter I highlight the historical and political awareness – particularly around colonialism's legacies – that did exist among some research participants. How responders related to historical entanglements of care and violence had direct implications for how they understood care, as well as how they conceived of and practised medical care during the Ebola epidemic. The wake influenced the response but only a few interviewees were able to articulate this. In this section I relate one interviewee's understanding of the conflation between care and violence, which shaped some Sierra Leoneans' hesitancy to seek care during the early stages of the epidemic.

Beyond Black Studies, and emerging out of an adjacent intellectual tradition, Piepzna-Samarasinha (2016, p. 39) explains that queer (and/ or) of colour, disabled 'people's fear of accessing care didn't come out of nowhere. It came out of generations and centuries where needing care meant being locked up, losing your human and civil rights, and being subject to abuse.' Reading Piepzna-Samarasinha and Theri Alice Pickens (2019), among other Black and Brown, Queer and non-binary disability justice thinkers, writers and activists, opens the door for sustained questionings and criticisms of how to think and practise care. Reading them alongside Black Studies writings on institutional care and care as violence also points to global similarities in experiences of institutional care where Black, Brown and Indigenous people are concerned. As Pickens (2019, p. 29) writes: 'the relationship between Blackness and disability writ large, is a relationship sutured at times by its connections, but also turned in and turned out by missed connections, erasures, and gaps'.

These connections, erasures and gaps are rooted in white supremacy and in the prescriptive upholding of heteronormative, cisgendered, middle-class, able, white bodies. They extend not only to how to live and experience disease and illness, but also to how to accept and receive care. Care, these experiences teach us, is sometimes justifiably resisted, encountered with suspicion and fled from. As with many of the writings I draw on here, the above are geographically anchored in the Americas, but the conflations between care and violence, and the resulting hesitancy to seek care, also manifested during the EVD epidemic in Sierra Leone.

In their writing, Piepzna-Samarasinha (2016) moves from an entanglement between care and state violence to care as state violence. That care can be violence is visible in the history of Sierra Leone at least twice: after the abolition of the British slave trade in 1807 when the British Navy intercepted slave ships off the coast of West Africa and resettled freed slaves in Sierra Leone, where they were enrolled in schemes of unpaid labour as 'apprentices' (Fyfe, 1962; Olusoga, 2016; see chapter 1 this volume). The apprenticeship scheme upheld a regime of servitude from which the enslaved had officially just been freed. The motivation for this, as I have detailed previously, was 'British care and philanthropy'. The second instance is what Frenkel and Western (1988) have described as 'humanitarian imperialism', wherein British colonisation of Sierra Leone was understood to be for the benefit and development of local populations. The historical overlap between discourses of care and the colonial violence that I have analysed with regard to infectious disease control in colonial Sierra Leone further speaks to care and its entanglement with antiblackness. In the aftermath of care as colonial violence, thinking care is about remembering and tending to Black death in the past and in the present, and considering the continuity of colonialism, the wake.

Thus to think care in our global postcolonial context is to remember its use as violence. In other words, the reality of the wake includes a past entanglement of care and violence or 'care as violence'. The majority of my interviewees did not consider how past experiences of violence could influence the behaviours of Sierra Leonean communities during the Ebola epidemic. For most, antiblackness and the colonial past were disregarded in their narrations of the response and of care practices. A few interviewees, however, did mention the colonial past. James, a white British doctor who had worked at Connaught Hospital spoke about the entanglements of violence and care. He acknowledged the reality of working in the wake of historical conflations of care and violence (albeit not in those terms). In his interview he referred to the hold that past experiences of violence have on Sierra Leonean attitudes to seeking medical care:

> I don't know if it's a true story but I was told, I think Siaka Stevens as president got a doctor to kill someone in his government, so you know … and there was a belief that this [the Ebola epidemic] was a US military experiment, well [the] US army had a research station at Kenema looking at viral haemorrhagic fevers, so these rumours are not sort of … they often have a seed of truth and reality was pretty far-fetched as well. So I don't feel dismissive or blame people for having these beliefs and what's really sad is that a lot of the time they were desperately trying to do what they thought was the right thing to do for their families and we were, the response saw them as a problem and they were acting out of compassion and sacrifice and heroism and that, that I find hard.

James recognised that Sierra Leone's historical and political landscape played an important role in shaping individual and communal attitudes to government and international care institutions. Medical care is here associated with violence, both in the belief that a Sierra Leonean president had used a doctor to kill someone, but also in the belief that the medical research conducted by Americans in the east of Sierra Léone was at the origin of the epidemic and, consequently, thousands of deaths. Importantly, James acknowledged that rumours on Ebola were based on historical and present realities. He recognised the reality of the epidemic occurring in the wake of violence. Here care's entanglement with state and/or institutional violence is a reality that needs to be acknowledged in the management of the response. Speaking about community perceptions of associating institutional care with violence he continued:

> the person seems certainly healthy, they're being dragged away by persons in space suits and then they all end up dead, and I think this is another thing that they experienced before. And you know what's more unrealistic? The truth? Or their belief? Actually, the truth sounds pretty far-fetched if you don't come from a biomedical tradition.

Again, James's statement attests to the hold that past violence has on present perceptions of care. His statement 'this is a thing they experienced before' echoed another statement he made during the course of our interview. Speaking of the east of Sierra Leone, where the epidemic first entered the country and where the first treatment centres were set up (MSF established an ETC in Kailahun District in June 2014) he said: 'People did not in the east trust foreigners you know and there's lots of historical reasons why that is understandable.'[2]

James cared about these realities, even if they were not his own because they shaped the lives (and deaths) of his patients and influenced the extent to which he could provide biomedical care. He also acknowledged that biomedical care's entanglements with histories and past experiences of violence were not considered in the response.

> I think that was a challenge from […] some of the Sierra Leonean and international leadership who did not have enough insights and I think particularly when it came to understandings of death and burials, [you] know people would just say 'Why are these people so crazy? Why are they putting their lives at risk for the sake of a burial?' It just doesn't seem to make sense. I think only when I started to understand the belief among some Sierra Leoneans about the afterlife and haunted afterlife and [that] there is actually worse things than death. 'There's worse things than death' – that is not something that exists in my view of the

world. Without understanding that – and I think there was a general lack of empathy of really putting ourselves in their shoes and asking the right questions about those things. And I think we did learn those lessons, but too late.

In James's account two meanings of care are present. On the one hand he attests to care's entanglement with historical violence and, while he does not centre the antiblackness that has characterised colonial and slave-trading violence in Sierra Leone, he acknowledges how past experiences of violence shaped Sierra Leonean communities' responses to institutional care during the Ebola epidemic. On the other hand, James's awareness of his patients' realities, that their reality of the epidemic differed from his, that their care needs differed from his conceptualisations of care, corresponds to Piepzna-Samarasinha's (2016, p. 40) invitation to 'turn on its head the model that disabled people can only passively receive care, not give it or determine what kind of care we want'. Similarly, we need to recognise the right of formerly colonised populations to not be receptive to models of institutionalised biomedical care former colonial powers have imposed on them previously. This is especially important in emergency situations such as epidemics. Maybe, thinking about care differently – recognising the politics and histories of care – can help us think and practise care beyond Western universalising conceptions of biomedicine. To care about Black life means recognising the reality of the wake and of past violence and their hold on the Ebola epidemic and response, even if antiblackness remains hard to grasp. To respect someone else's reality without fully understanding it can be a leap of faith, but it is one that we owe Black, African and formerly colonised people, especially if we are to combat the spectre of biomedicine's antiblack past. A focus on this analytical and political hold warrants a centring of perspectives, rather than enactments (Mol, 2002) and an effort to care beyond the objective unembodied realities of Ebola-related care that Mol invites.

Rethinking the Human

To care about Black life, medically during the EVD epidemic and conceptually, necessitated an understanding of the historical entanglements of biomedical care and institutional/state violence. A number of studies have explored the question of trust and mistrust in the context of EVD in either Sierra Leone or the more recent outbreaks in DRC in North Kivu and Ituri in 2018–20 and I have referenced some of them in this book (i.e. Lipton, 2017; see also Richards et al., 2019 or Vinck et al., 2019). However, as Richardson et al. (2019, p. 1) have also pointed out, studies which focus on issues of trust and mistrust in communities affected with Ebola and people's suspicion of/reluctance to seek biomedical care, without addressing the coloniality (and I would add antiblackness) that factors into these attitudes, 'too readily serve as a smokescreen that enables and perpetuates ongoing structural inequities – notably, by omitting consideration of global power relations, colonial history and contemporary extractive political economies'. To move beyond understandings of Ebola epidemics centred on the trust/mistrust dichotomy, centring coloniality and antiblackness in our thinking about the provision of biomedical care necessitates a rethinking of the human, in other words, an engagement with how global/public health, natural sciences and medical sciences in particular think about the human as divorced from the conceptual politics that made it. The idea of a universal shared humanity underlies and motivates much humanitarian action and intervention, and certainly played a role – alongside pre-existing colonial relations – in different states and NGOs contributing to the setting up of the Sierra Leonean Ebola response. The biological groundings of this shared humanity seem self-evident. Humans share 99 per cent of their genetic make-up (NHGRI, 2018) – a scientific argument often brought forward to argue against the idea of *race*. However, as Jamaican theorist and writer Sylvia Wynter (2001; see also Ferreira da Silva, 2015) has written, such biological groundings need to be examined carefully. As she explains, the birth of European secular ontological Man went hand in hand with colonial expansion and the conceptualisation of what it means to be human has long been colonised by Europe.

The move from a European belief system based on shared Christian values from which a shared humanity could be derived was put into question following early European imperialism. During early voyages and the discovery of the Americas, so Wynter (2003), Europeans were confronted with human beings who did not share their belief in a Christian God. European epistemic categorisation of the meaning of the human thus pivoted from an ontology based on universal Christianity, to one based on universal biology. This principle still underlies how we think about and define the human. However, Wynter urges us to question the parameters of this universal biology and the political work it performs. As Walter Mignolo (2015, p. 108) writes:

Wynter refuses to embrace the entity of the Human independently of the epistemic categories and concepts that created it by suggesting instead that our conceptualizations of the Human are produced within an autopoietic system. The problem of the Human is thus not identity-based per se but in the enunciations of what it means to be Human – enunciations that are concocted and circulated by those who most convincingly (and powerfully) imagine the 'right' or 'noble' or 'moral' characteristics of Human and in this project their own image-experience of the Human into the sphere of Universal Humanness. The Human is therefore the product of a particular epistemology, yet it appears to be (and is accepted as) a naturally independent entity existing in the world.

Wynter's work can help us think through conceptualisations of care in relation to the international Ebola response in Sierra Leone. Discussions around Sierra Leoneans' reluctance to seek biomedical care or their insistence on holding traditional burials, discussed by James in the previous section, were largely seen as irrational and complicating international (white European) efforts to stem the spread of EVD. The provision of (biomedical) care rested and relied on a specific vision of what it means to be human. In this case, wanting to live and be cured by biomedical means more than caring for the dead or the living, even if this meant likely infection.[3] The conceptualisation of the human that underlay these critiques was based on a set of human behaviours deemed rational and universal. When behaviours diverged from these expectations the response resorted to more militaristic means to fold Sierra Leoneans into the parameters of the biomedical response.

Mignolo (2015, p. 108) further explains:

> Wynter's writings demonstrate that Western epistemology built itself on a concept of Human and Humanity that, in turn, served to legitimate the epistemic foundation that created it. That is, Human and Humanity were created as the enunciated that projects and propels to universality the local image of the enunciator. The enunciator assumes, and thus postulates, that his concept of Human and Humanity is valid for every human being on the planet.

Biomedical regimes and humanitarian interventions are built on this local image of the human *propelled to universality*. Notably, Wynter critiques the biological grounding the universal human subject was imbued with.

Rather than biology and the natural sciences more broadly being an objective depiction and analysis of the world, Wynter (2003) sees them as yet another discursive and political product which, in the case of the question of what it means to be human, was used by European thinkers to naturalise colonial hierarchies and relations through the invention of *race* (Ferreira da Silva, 2015). The biological norm has long been modelled on white European able-bodied men. European Man, according to Wynter, is over-represented in our understanding of the Human, both politically and biologically. The idea of race then, and within it specifically the idea of Blackness, serves to establish hierarchies within and in relation to the idea of shared universal biological humanity. What discourses around care and care politics during EVD epidemics reveal, is that even without naming Blackness, people of African descent in Sierra Leone, or the DRC during the 2018–20 epidemic, had their humanity questioned precisely because they at times refused the offers of biomedical care conceived on the basis of a shared biological humanity. Existing analyses have failed to acknowledge that these care regimes and the conceptions of the human that underlay them are based on the over-representation of white European Man and did not take the coloniality of care and biomedicine into account.

Practising Care: The Spatial Management of Risk and its Racialisation

The Ontopolitics of Ebola

I continue with a focus on Ebola care practices and the spatial (and to a lesser extent temporal) management of risk of infection, and ultimately death from infection with EVD. Following Mol (2002) and drawing on interviews with medical responders working in a variety of makeshift and purpose-built Ebola treatment centres and holding units I analyse how Ebola's ontologies were enacted as condition and as process. Then, drawing on Alexander Weheliye's (2015) writings on racialising assemblages, I further conceptualise how the risk of infection was managed spatially, and how the way in which Ebola's ontologies are enacted contributed to their racialisation. I argue that how Ebola IPC (infection prevention and control) was enacted, shaped the organisation of ETCs and EHUs (Ebola holding units) spatially and reinforced pre-existing, yet rarely openly acknowledged, hierarchies in humanity as discussed by Wynter (2001, 2003) and built on by Weheliye (2015).

Weheliye's (2015) work draws on Black feminist literature to interrogate dominant discourses on race and biopolitics. His concept of racialising assemblages (2015, p. 4) stipulates that rather than race being a biological or cultural category, it is 'a set of socio-political processes that discipline humanity into full humans, not-quite humans, and nonhumans'. He argues (2015, p. 3):

> If racialization is understood not as a biological or cultural descriptor but as a conglomerate of sociopolitical relations that discipline humanity into full humans, not-quite-humans, and nonhumans, then blackness designates a changing system of unequal power structures that apportion and delimit which humans can lay claim to full human status and which humans cannot. Conversely, 'white supremacy may be understood as a logic of social organisation that produces regimented, institutionalized, and militarized conceptions of hierarchized "human" difference.'[4]

In ETCs such hierarchies of human difference are reproduced, highly regimented and institutionalised. The spatial organisation of Ebola treatment centres; their classification and distribution of patients into different zones according to their infection status does several things: (1) it illustrates Weheliye's racialising assemblages and (2) it aligns with Ruth Wilson Gilmore's (2002, p. 261) definition of racism as 'the state-sanctioned and/ or extra-legal production and exploitation of group-differentiated vulnerabilities to premature death in distinct yet densely interconnected political geographies'. This spatial organisation and the accompanying categorisation of patients meant that anyone infected with EVD who entered an ETC was integrated into a unidirectional flow system, which moved patients from a green to a red zone or from suspected to confirmed to dead or recovered. For healthcare workers whose care practices were shaped by the constant possibility of infection and subsequent death, infection meant re-entering this flow as a patient. In Sierra Leone, 0.11 per cent of the general population died from EVD in comparison to 6.85 per cent of Sierra Leonean healthcare workers (Evans et al., 2015). Though for international staff the numbers were radically different (several contracted Ebola but survived after receiving treatment in Europe, and two Spanish priests died after caring for Ebola patients at the very beginning of the epidemic), death was – especially at the beginning of the epidemic – omnipresent.

This 'possibility of always-imminent death' (Sharpe, 2016) was in ETCs and EHUs localised and managed through flows that reinforced the difference between those living (and moving) and those consigned to the red zones (confirmed wards) alongside the 'human – not-quite human – nonhuman axis', identified by Weheliye (2015). In contrast to biopolitics, critiqued by Weheliye (2015, p. 8) for its failure to acknowledge that 'there exists no portion of the modern human that is not subject to racialisation', racialising assemblages accepts that variations in our experience of being human have long been artificially tied to phenotype. I superimpose the hierarchy of humanness that Weheliye (2015) draws attention to, on the spatial trajectory of EVD patients in which admission to an ETC started a journey towards either an affirmation of humanity (life) or non-humanity (death). Here the wake manifests once again along racial lines in that, for IPC reasons, Black patients were distributed according to aforementioned spatial categories whereas white staff, whose narrations I draw on here, could move freely through the centre and were often in charge of patient and staff flows.

Mol (2002, p. 104), writing about the enactment of atherosclerosis in Hospital Z in the Netherlands, notes that atherosclerosis exists both as process and as condition. Writing about the reality of the disease for vascular surgeons and internists she writes:

Here, atherosclerosis is enacted as a present condition, there, as a process that has a history. Tensions between these ways to enact the reality of the disease are articulated. But it does not come to a full-blown fight. Instead, the differences between the condition atherosclerosis and the atherosclerotic process are distributed.

The tensions that arise due to the multiplicity of atherosclerosis, according to Mol (2002), do not escalate because they are spatially distributed between the outpatient department and the department of internal medicine. Similar distributions structured Ebola's ontopolitics during the international response in Sierra Leone, albeit in a more restricted space. The spatial dimensions of ETCs and EHUs allowed for some degree of distribution of Ebola as condition and Ebola as process, but on a smaller scale than was the case in Mol's (2002) case study of Hospital Z. Whether treatment units were located in existing hospitals or were purpose-built, they were generally separated into zones with increasing risk of infection: the green zone, the orange zone and the red zone, with the latter housing confirmed patients in various stages of progression of the disease. These spatial zones structured the material practices of Ebola care. Dina and Maria, two epidemiologists who worked in different purpose-built ETCs both spoke to this in separate interviews and how these zones shaped their practices spatially and materially:

> *Dina* [indicating map – Figure 11]: Here that would be the green zone, meaning low risk, so you would have to wash your hands. And we [epidemiologists] were in the orange zone, so the kind of thing that is not the wards is orange [...] and the red zone is inside the wards, but the clinic is orange [suspected cases] with like super high risk. So you would have to go in PPE in the red zone. We had scrubs for the orange zone.

> *Maria*: As the epidemiologist we were not allowed to go in the red zone so [...] the patient would have to be ambulatory to be able to [...] do the interview so we would be in the orange zone and we would have the distance between us like the 3, 4 metres and through the distance we would talk to the patient and use a simplified questionnaire to see who the contacts were. [...] And these we would then transmit to the local authorities [...] and there was another organisation responsible for the contact tracing.

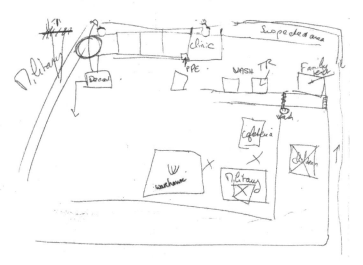

Figure 11   Map of ETC drawn from memory by Dina. The red zone is in the top left corner, left of the clinic. The 'white worker treatment centre', which Dina spoke about in chapter 1, is in the bottom right corner designated 'Military'. (Photo by the author)

Several things are worth noting here. As epidemiologists, Dina and Maria are not directly involved in patient care and their movements are thus constricted to the green and orange zones. They do not enter the red zone in which risk of infection is highest. Even when interacting with patients they do not cross into the red zone. The spatial distance between themselves and suspected and confirmed cases becomes one of the cornerstones shaping their movements, as well as how they can do their work, how they obtain their data and what they wear. In Maria's account, Ebola is both a condition that determines which patients she interacts with ('so I was in contact [...] with only [...] the cases that were suspects and then negatives of course') and a process that needs to be interrupted through contact tracing.

Both epidemiologists, when speaking about the disease in their work, spoke about it as a condition or, in their words, 'status'. Describing her daily work to me, Dina said the following:

So [I was] basically trying to collect data about patients there and trying to create a database and follow the epidemic. [...] so I was entering data, and if they [the forms] were missing data I would go back to the clinicians and [...] so I was basically checking if they had lab results and what was the Ebola status, [pauses] it was supposed to be positive. Yeah and I was chasing data about their Ebola status, what were the symptoms and things like that. And chasing that the clinicians were actually filling [in] the forms.

For Dina, Ebola is a status and specifically a positive status on a form that comes in with the patient, is filled in by the doctor (but not always) and then transformed into data by her. What Dina describes is a process of transforming Ebola from one (or multiple) thing(s) into another. Her statement 'I was chasing data about their Ebola status, what were the symptoms and things like that' indicates the multiplicity inherent in turning Ebola from a list of possible symptoms into a status, to translate several things into one. In Dina's case all patients who arrived at the treatment centre were supposed to have a positive status, but her subsequent description ('I was chasing data about their Ebola status [...] and chasing the clinicians') indicates that obtaining a clear status was at times difficult. At the same time, her statement also shows the tensions for practice in Ebola's enactment. For clinicians filling in a form, according to Dina, seemed secondary to catering to other elements of the ontologies of

Ebola, such as administering pain medications (pain) or cleaning or feeding patients (vomiting, bleeding, diarrhoea and dehydration). For Dina, obtaining these forms constituted the basis of her work and allowed her to 'follow the epidemic'. Following the epidemic took different forms of practice. While Dina did this through the forms and data available to her on a computer, contact tracers, who Maria mentioned above, followed the disease in the community.

Having a negative or positive Ebola status became one of the cornerstones of the way treatment centres operated and organised patients along a hierarchy of human difference in relation to EVD and, given the disease's high mortality rate, the possibility of imminent death (Sharpe, 2016). As Dina stated above, only patients with positive Ebola results were admitted into the centre in which she worked. Simultaneously as Maria and Dina's descriptions of treatment centre zones indicate, Ebola status also shaped the spatial arrangements of treatment centres and units. The difference between a positive or negative status had important repercussions on mobility in the centre, with positive statuses confined to the red zones. However, in the status too, we can find tension. Laura, a British doctor who worked as medical director in various treatment centres described the Ebola testing process to me:

Testing-wise we used to get results usually that night but we faced a lot of opposition from a man who was running the lab at the time and he would often refuse to do our 72 [hours] repeat samples on people who initially tested negative and we'd have to really fight for it. We weren't getting CT values or anything like that we just got a positive or negative.[5] There were some interesting things happening like we had a guy referred to us at one point who, he was a doctor, had potentially been exposed in his hospital, where there had been several healthcare worker infections. He didn't really have many symptoms, but he had some low-level symptoms so they tested him and they tested him on a Monday, they called him on a Monday to inform him his test was negative. They called me on the Wednesday to inform me that his test was positive and he was coming to us. So, when he arrived he said to me – I didn't know that part – he just said to me 'Tell me, is my test now positive or …?' and I said 'I don't know but what I've been told is it is positive' and I called the lab or our lab tech several times to speak to the lab and I was told no it's definitely positive.

In Laura's account the simple binary of an Ebola status, so important in structuring the spatial organisation of treatment centres and units, gets complicated and turned into a contested reality. A result is first negative and then positive. Due to the absence of CT values, which indicate a numeric continuum, not a positive or negative status, Laura could not be sure whether this was a low or a high positive value. Here Ebola is a continuum, rather than a binary of negative and positive, green or red zone. At the same time, the tension here partially stems from the personal politics that characterised the treatment centre's relationship with the laboratory running their tests. Laura's statements 'we faced a lot of opposition from the guy running the lab', 'we'd have to really fight for it' indicate tension of a different nature, not due to different enactments of the disease but caused by outside factors.

When we spoke, Laura had come up with an explanation for the inconsistency in test results:

> But I think what happened at that point because of the management at [laboratory] being a problem [...] I think maybe they were reviewing previous results and they probably went 'That's positive' and it maybe was a low-level positive, so yeah and so we admitted this guy to our confirmed ward but we didn't really know what to do because he wasn't sick so we gave him a mask and some gloves, he was a doctor, we basically said 'do not help anyone, do not touch anything if you can avoid it' and you know he never became any more symptomatic with us, he didn't have a fever. We tested him again three days later and he was negative and we discharged him.

Laura is able to explain the tension in the lab result through problems in management at the laboratory. In her analysis the result's ambiguity is brought about through inconsistencies in laboratory practice. In Mol's (2002) account tension is distributed geographically in Hospital Z, here tensions between the lab and the clinic collide and disrupt the spatial segregation of treatment zones. The patient is admitted to the confirmed ward, but told not to touch anything. The accuracy of his Ebola status is in doubt. The spatial zone (the confirmed ward/red zone) that the patient is committed to does coincide with his lab result but not his symptoms. As Laura describes 'he never became any more symptomatic with us'. Despite Laura's hesitation ('we didn't really know what to do') and her affirmation that 'he wasn't sick', the patient is sent to the confirmed ward in which patients in various stages of EVD are cared for and in which the risk of infection is highest. The patient is placed with those whose vulnerability to death from EVD is highest.

Laura's account also gives an insight into the hierarchy of medical evidence at work here. In this example, laboratory test results (in the form of numbers based on the patient's viral load) are translated into a condition and trump bodily evidence ('he never became any more symptomatic with us') and Laura's professional assessment that 'he wasn't sick'. The disease's laboratory status cancels out the patient's symptoms, or lack thereof, and also his entitlement to be in a ward more distant to one with a high chance of infection, such as the suspect ward. Here, the realities of EVD are hierarchical with Ebola as positive or negative status at the top. This leads to a higher risk of infection for the patient than if Laura's assessment or his bodily symptoms were at the top of the epistemic hierarchy. Laura knows this but abides by the hierarchy. In this example, Ebola is enacted in two ways, not only in two different locations, but in one body, whose lab results produce a (seemingly temporary, low-level) positive Ebola status without returning corresponding bodily symptoms.

Care as Flow

Ebola care is subjected to spatial and temporal rhythms. Spatial and temporal flows are an integral part of working in an ETC or EHU. In medical terms, flow is the regulation of patient and staff movements through the hospital or treatment unit for purposes of patient and staff safety from nosocomial infection (infections occurring in hospitals). Flow was an integral part of Ebola care practices and shaped the way in which staff interacted with the geography and built environment of the treatment centres or units. Tom, a British doctor working in Connaught Hospital during the outbreak, described flow as one of the basic components of setting up effective Ebola care ('Safety around Ebola units requires a couple of things. One of them is – the appreciation of flow'). Maria, the epidemiologist, quoted earlier, described the flow that shaped the rhythm of work in the unit in which she worked. She based this flow largely on an understanding of Ebola as a condition (or status) that is either positive or negative:

> So there was a whole circle, a patient flow depending on the first outcome of the test. People would come to the emergency wards, they

would be seen there by the health professionals, then if they would be admitted based on their admission criteria they would move into the suspect area. They would wait there until confirmation came, if they were negative they would either stay there if we couldn't transfer them into the hospital or they would be moved if they were confirmed into the confirmed area.

Here flows enact a treatment centre in which distances and spaces work to navigate the possibility of infection and death. Each movement that Maria describes, from patient arrival at the hospital, to testing, to suspect and possibly confirmed areas moves the patient along a spatial and ontological trajectory closer to or away from the possibility of death and humanity.

Laura, quoted earlier, described the organisation of flow in the treatment centre in which she worked. Her account reifies Ebola as a status, but also attests to the possibility of infection and death inherent in flow management:

We made it very clear at the beginning of every day that the only way into the treatment facility was through the door of suspects from donning [putting PPE on] and the only way out was through doffing [taking PPE off] and that we had a unilateral flow through the unit which meant you went from suspect to confirmed and you never went back again. We did have an exit from suspect, so if we had a patient in suspect who tested negative twice we could take them out through suspect without having to go through confirmed, and we had a sort of a shower cubicle outside of suspect, well not outside, outside the ward, but still within the high-risk zone where we could wash them down before taking them out and it was basically out the triage exit, and we tried to keep that area sprayed clean with chlorine all the time if someone had come through there. If there were any spills [of bodily fluid] we treated them with chlorine and absorbing matters, we were following MSF protocols.

Laura's description indicates the importance of movement in the conception of treatment centres and units and the spatialisation of the possibility of always-imminent death (Sharpe, 2016). As with green, orange and red zones, the flow established in the refurbished hospital in which Laura worked, operated to confine the possibility of death to certain spaces. These spaces overlapped with the confirmed or suspect zones or wards, whose demarcation was based on Ebola as condition. Simultaneously, the passages from zones in which death was imminent and those where it became more distant were clearly marked and demarcated through practice and materials. The patients' proximity to death is regulated and enacted through their movement through the treatment centre. Chlorine kept the exit from the suspect area clean from bodily spills. She continued:

> If a patient was deceased their body was decontaminated with chlorine and then they were placed in a wrap and then in a heavy-duty body bag although we didn't have those at the beginning in [hospital 1], they weren't available for a bit of time but we would decontaminate them, wrap them in this sort of shroud, and then put them in the heavy-duty body bag, or some form of plastic body bag and carry them out to the morgue.

A shroud, heavy-duty or plastic body bag were the materials used to confine and demarcate death. Here, IPC measures extend beyond the death of a patient. Given that Ebola patients are most infectious at the time of and shortly after their death, when their viral load is highest, the patient's dead body is subjected to similar spatial and mobile constraints as the patient was in life. If anything, those constraints are intensified materially and spatially to ensure the reduction of risk of infection. The dead body leaves the realm of always-imminent death but not through the same exits or routes taken by those living. In the spatial dynamics of IPC, racialising assemblages (Weheliye, 2015) are enacted spatially and reinforce a colonial-racial hierarchy in which Black life is tethered ever more closely to the possibility of always-imminent death (Sharpe, 2016). EVD strips bodies of their humanness, even in death, in which they are denied sharing a space with the uninfected dead and are buried in non-traditional ways.

In some instances, this link between movement and death or life was enacted nominally too. Describing the flow system, Tom stated:

> *Tom*: So the flow from clean to dirty or what is sometimes called green to red zone. So creating a flow, which means that you need normally free doorways, you know, free entry points, so one is an entry for staff from the clean zone, one is an exit for staff from the patient area and one is a dirty exit which is where either corpses or Ebola-positive patients come out of.
>
> *Lioba*: And it's called dirty exit?
>
> *Tom*: Ahm, no, I guess that's in my head. In my head you got a clean exit and a dirty exit.

Tom's description both speaks to the importance of regimented flows through an ETC or EHU for general safety and reveals how safety from infection was linked to the built environment. In order for EVD care to take place in a safe environment (in other words to guard carers against the possibility of Ebola death), movement through that environment had to be carefully planned and the environment at times adjusted by freeing door-ways or changing the layout of existing wards. His account also speaks to the way in which movement through the treatment centre or holding unit marked patients and staff as distinct groups. Ebola's contagiousness led to the segregation and directionality of movements. Patients moved through the treatment centre or unit in ways that were different from staff. At the same time, the directionality of movements was also imbued with mean-ing. Tom's description 'the flow from clean to dirty' resonates with Laura's description of the unidirectionality of flows. In both instances, the fur-ther a patient or member of staff moved along established flows through the treatment unit, the closer they came to the possibility of death and to inhabiting that dual space of Blackness and non-humanness (Weheliye, 2015). As a consequence, these differentiated movements enacted Ebola as contagious and deathly possibility in Black bodies.

As Tom's and Laura's accounts show, movement and flow were imbued with meaning and signalled one's progression from human, to not-quite human to non-human or dead. They also illustrate how one group's vulner-ability to premature death (Gilmore, 2002) was enacted spatially in order to protect healthcare staff and patients. There is ambiguity here, and the discomfort that arises from living in a global world shaped by antiblack-ness in which we already aren't afforded the luxury of all the options and have to contend with the reproduction of Black vulnerability. Simultane-ously, flows could also be life-affirming. Laura explained the procedure for discharging patients who had tested negative twice:

If we were going in that day, we wouldn't check on any other patient, we'd go straight to the patient we were discharging so we hadn't contam-inated ourselves and then discharge them and then discharge another if there was more than one, and then dress them in clean clothes that we'd also brought in with us.

Here, changes in flow and material signal survival. The usual flow is inter-rupted to protect the life of the patient who is about to be discharged. Clean clothes are brought in from the green or clean zone to signal the patient's imminent passage back to life. At the same time, Laura's statement 'so we hadn't contaminated ourselves' indicates the high association between patients' bodies and risk of infection, and the careful spatial and practical planning that characterised Ebola care and made it sustainable.

Ebola care was not only subjected to spatial flows and zones, but also to temporal ones. The flows throughout the wards, from suspect to confirmed patients, had to be carried out in full PPE, as lighter PPE and scrubs were only allowed in the green zones. Due to local weather conditions this limited the time that staff could spend on rounds through the ETC or EHU. Time spent attending to patients in the confirmed ward varied from treatment centre to treatment centre but interviewees reported they would on average spend between one and three hours in the red zone in full PPE. Jack and Hector, two British doctors who both worked in purpose-built facilities, stated that they spent between 45 minutes and one hour in the red zone on each round. In Laura's case this was different. She stated:

> We had the white suits at the beginning and we weren't supposed to be in for longer than an hour and a half in the white suits. Then we became increasingly concerned by the white suits [...] so then we moved to the yellow suits and then we said you shouldn't be in for longer than an hour. But I think I was probably in a white suit at one point for just under three hours and I was probably in a yellow suit for at least two if not more hours.

PPE, in conjunction with the weather conditions in which Ebola care was practised contributed to determining the temporal rhythms of Ebola care. This had implications for how care was given and what responders felt they were able to do without putting themselves at risk. Laura and her team moved from lighter white suits to heavier yellow suits, which decreased the time they were able to actively care for patients on the confirmed ward. Anne, a British nurse who worked as the medical lead in two ETCs, described the implications of spatial and temporal regiments for Ebola care:

> The care that you would give people in terms of frequency of cleaning them isn't what you would want ideally because people would just be cleaned like when you went in and not in between [...]. I remember once there was a young girl and, just as we had to leave the red zone

'cause our time was up, and it was like a hot day, she fell onto the floor, but we couldn't really stay to help her back on, so she just had to stay there until the next people went in.

Anne's regret at the altered standard of care and her team's decision to leave the girl lying on the floor does not negate the reality of violence and biomedical care as violence that characterised aspects of working in Ebola treatment centres and that is centred in BIPOC (Black, Indigenous and other People of Colour) analyses of disabilities and care (Piepzna-Samarasinha, 2016; Pickens, 2019). Anne's quote also indicates how, for clinical staff, Ebola was enacted in the realm of always-imminent death, and how care with violence became part of medical practice.

Care and (Shared) Risk

An antidote to care as violence is care as sharing risk (Sharpe, 2016, 2018). In Sharpe's work, sharing risk in the face of structural and epistemic violence constitutes an emotional and practical act of care. Sharing risk became important during the Sierra Leonean Ebola epidemic and the organisation of its response. Seeing shared risk as an element of care enables an analysis of care practice that is aware of and acts in spite of the possibility of imminent death which was present during the epidemic. In the interviews that I conducted, awareness of the possibility of imminent death was widespread. Awareness around the repetition of the wake was however largely sidelined.

Caring for Ebola patients, who effectively lived with the possibility of always-imminent death, meant embracing an element of shared risk; however, the level of risk depended on the treatment centre or holding unit those international responders worked in. Effectively, risk was not shared equally and was distributed along medical and postcolonial hierarchies. When medical responders spoke about their decision to travel to Sierra Leone and work on the Ebola epidemic, the risk they referred to mostly represented their own risk of infection, rather than someone else's risk. While some risks were shared with Sierra Leonean Ebola patients (risk of infection, risk of quarantine and, ultimately, risk of death), working in a (purpose-built) international treatment centre mitigated these risks considerably. Jack, a British doctor who worked in an international purpose-built facility in Sierra Leone, confirmed this:

We knew that in practice the people who were getting infected were non-healthcare workers caring for family, were healthcare workers doing out-of-hospital work, were healthcare workers in government healthcare facilities, you know that. Actually, people working in international facilities were generally not getting infected.

James, who worked at Connaught Hospital spoke to how risk was shared or not shared in his EHU:

A very legitimate point a lot of Sierra Leonean medical colleagues made was that I was likely to be medevac'd. Officially the British government told me we would not be medevac'd, explicitly we would not be, but we kind of thought that we might be. But we knew Sierra Leonean colleagues wouldn't and we knew what the outcomes would be for them, so ... and as much as we were facing – we were in the same PPE as our colleagues – and we were facing the same risk and it's a pretty deadly disease whether you are medevac'd or not, the fact that we knew we'd be medevac'd, was you know ...

James's account reveals the postcolonial hierarchies at work during the response and his awareness of them. His discussion of facing, yet not quite facing, the same risk as his Sierra Leonean medical colleagues speaks to their respective proximity to the possibility of infection and of death inside the EHU. James, who was relatively certain that him and his British colleagues would be medevac'd could navigate the risk of death differently than his Sierra Leonean colleagues. While the message in James's statement is clear, he finds himself unable to articulate the deadly consequences this colonial-racial inequality could have.

Jack spoke to how risk was distributed along medical hierarchies:

We also went out with lots of paramedics and the paramedics were terrific and by far my favourite staff group to have in the response. [...] They're much more used to dealing with personal risk, you know they're out in the community dealing with risk all the time, whereas we're [doctors] all ensconced in hospitals where we manage that much more effectively.

Different medical staff groups handled the risks involved in participating in the Ebola response in different ways. Jack's comparison of paramedics' and doctors' respective abilities to handle risk also indicates that care practices outside of a traditional hospital setting seemed to him more risk-prone than care practices occurring in hospitals, where he had experience working as a doctor. Here, spatial settings are differently imbued with risks. In a hospital, according to Jack, risks can be navigated more effectively than in the public, where the paramedics he encountered worked.

Ria, an Ebola response manager for a medical NGO, also spoke to the association between the care practices needed in the international response and different staff groups. Her statement placed a heavy emphasis on the necessity for care, as opposed to other work:

> There was a higher demand for nurses because there was no cure for Ebola and a lot of the work around Ebola was around cleaning, feeding, changing bed covers [...] So sending doctors was quite problematic, because [...] they're not trained in how to care for people.

Ria and Jack's comments emphasised that the work needed in Ebola treatment units was care work, that the risk of infection was high and that specific staff groups, such as paramedics and nurses, are generally associated with carrying out these types of work. More importantly, this risk was especially high outside of international, purpose-built ETCs and EHUs. Overall, risk seemed to operate along medical, spatial and postcolonial hierarchies and was distributed unequally among people involved in the response.

These hierarchical dynamics were somewhat lessened at Connaught Hospital. Among the people I interviewed who worked at Connaught, the hierarchies around care work that usually permeate medical practice were broken down. Gareth, a doctor who went out to work in Connaught Hospital, described the sharing of tasks (and risk) in the Ebola holding unit of Connaught:

> One person would be assessing patients for their suitability to be admitted to the unit, someone else would be going to the unit to make sure the people inside were ok, someone would be dealing with discharges, there was cleaning and cleaning of the patients and the room and dealing with dead bodies and administration of drugs, so all those tasks were split up between whoever was on the shift. [...] when you were working in the unit everyone was considered the same level [...].

The EHU of Connaught Hospital thus became a place in which medical hierarchies were, to a large degree, suspended. The practices described by Gareth (cleaning bodies, administering drugs, cleaning the room) were practices of medical care shared by other doctors and nurses working in the hospital. At the same time, Connaught was not a purpose-built facility. The spatial and resource constraints of Connaught considerably increased risks of infection. Here the flattening of medical hierarchies was accompanied by a heightened possibility of death for international and national staff in comparison to purpose-built facilities. Nevertheless, as James pointed out earlier, for his Sierra Leonean colleagues the risk of working with Ebola patients continued to be higher.

Alex, a doctor who volunteered at Connaught Hospital, illustrated how a specific incident at Connaught manifested as 'care as shared risk' (Sharpe, 2016) and how they conjured the possibility of imminent death by talking about the materials their care practice relied on. Alex told me about an incident that had happened when administering the drug diazepam intravenously in the EHU of Connaught Hospital. Diazepam, more commonly known as Valium, is a drug that, when administered at a low dosage, produces a calming effect; it is often used to treat anxiety and, when administered at a higher dosage, puts patients to sleep (ASHP and SCCM, 2002). The onset of diazepam's calming qualities differs, depending on the way it is being administered. Through oral administration, the effects materialise after between 20 and 40 minutes (Dym and Ogle, 2011). When administered intravenously (through an IV) the medication takes effect between 2 and 5 minutes (Jacobi et al., 2002). This information is important when analysing the incident that Alex recounted. Speaking about the atmosphere in the Ebola treatment unit and patients' fears, they told me how they injured themselves in the red zone, the area of Connaught Hospital's EHU, which is the most infectious area of the hospital:

It was a difficult choice where one of my patients was very unwell and quite delirious and agitated, and so what you want to do for the individual patient is sedate them so they can be more relaxed. [...] You want them to calm down and so what I wanted to do is give him some diazepam, but obviously with every additional intervention that you introduce into that red zone you put yourself at additional risk. But I had decided that it made sense and we had those little plastic things to open the vials with, but because the quality of the vials we got were quite poor, the distribution of the plastic, or actually of the glass across the vial was suboptimal and two people before me had gotten this same injury in the red zone. So I broke off the cap and the cap itself was very thick and even though I used all the right protective gear, the vial itself crushed in my fingers and went through three pairs of gloves and pierced my finger in the red zone.

Alex, like the other responders I quoted, spoke about risk, although they linked it more directly to medical practice and specifically to caring for their patient. The decision to administer the medication intravenously can be interpreted as, on the one hand signifying a high level of care, due to the much faster onset of diazepam's calming effects, or, on the other hand, it could be conditioned by the progress the disease had made in the patient, rendering him 'unwell', 'quite delirious' and 'agitated', which possibly meant he was not able to swallow the medication, when administered orally. The patient and the patient's body and mental state shape and motivate Alex's practice. Their next words 'obviously with every additional intervention that you introduce into that red zone you put yourself at additional risk' show that Alex understood that calming their patient and making him feel 'more relaxed' directly increased their risk of exposure as does their admission 'But I had decided that it made sense'. As in Sharpe's (2016) accounts of shared risk, Alex cared for this patient in an environment in which care came with increased risks and accepted the risk of infection to ease their patient's suffering. Alex's description of how the injury itself occurred is suggestive of the ontopolitics of Ebola care (and the concomitant risk) in Connaught Hospital during the outbreak. In their account, risk of infection is enacted through the practice of opening a vial containing diazepam. It materialises through low-quality materials, the preceding occurrences of this injury linked to the particular practice of opening this type of vial and the protective measure of wearing three pairs of gloves to protect oneself against infection.

As in Mol's (2002) account of atherosclerosis, Ebola is never one thing, but rather appears in materials and practices. The way Alex speaks about the incident indicates that the quality of the materials in use did not compare to the standard of materials in medical practice that they were used to. While Mol's (2002) writings on the multiple ontologies of atherosclerosis take an in-depth look at the materiality of medical practice, the tensions she describes arise from a multiplicity of materials and practices and the realities they produce, not from low-quality materials, as is the case in Connaught Hospital. Similarly, Alex's description of the vial's shards piercing through three pairs of gloves speaks to the specificity of medical practices during an Ebola response. The additional material barrier between the Ebola virus and an as yet uninfected organism that is provided by two extra pairs of gloves enacts Ebola as highly infectious, but also points to the disease's exceptional nature, which requires material distance through improvised barriers. The risk of infection is not only the result of the virus, but results from the structural and material contexts of postcolonial Sierra Leone. Risk is here enacted as something that is close by, ubiquitous and against which the body of the doctor should ideally be 'ensconced'.

Alex continued to speak about this experience by linking it to the broader context of working in, what they called, 'a makeshift unit', as opposed to a purpose-built facility:

> We hadn't checked before we started to make sure the correct concentration of chlorine was available where it should be and it wasn't and so what you should do in that scenario is immediately submerge your hand into the chlorine, but we had to first mix it up, we couldn't find the things … we tried to work with the hospital management and the supply, so like soap [laughs] and gloves and just simple basic things like that […] so the hospital would get supplies from like a national [centre], I can't remember what they're called, it is part of the government and they would disperse like medications or whatever. So there were all these delays and you know of that particular injury, the two people who'd been exposed before me one had got Ebola and one hadn't and so, like yeah that could have happened in any of the other units, but also working in a makeshift unit, where everything isn't working as perfect as you would want it means you're at higher risk of those kinds of things happening.

Alex's continued description of this incident further reveals the materiality of Ebola care in an emergency setting. Chlorine, which, as I have written in chapter 1, was at times perceived as deadly by members of the community, is here, in its concentrated and liquid form in a bucket in the red zone of Connaught Hospital, a sought-after remedy. At the same time, its remedying characteristics, as Alex describes, depend on the correct concentration and placement of chlorine and its availability in the correct location. In Alex's account, the risk of infection, the unavailability of materials and the low-quality of tools all contribute to making the possibility of infection and death from infection more probable. In the red zone, Sharpe's (2016) 'possibility of always-imminent death' is spatialised.

Alex also makes an important point about the spatial arrangements in which their care, and the Ebola care of the hospital took place. Their analysis of the incident ('that could have happened in any of the other units, but also working in a makeshift unit, where everything isn't working as perfect as you would want it') places their comments on the absence of correctly mixed chlorine and low-quality vials in a political context. One of the reasons the risks of working in Connaught Hospital, a government hospital, were higher was because of the lower quality of materials available from local supply chains. Miki, one of the British IPC nurses working at the hospital, and I had the following exchange with regard to Connaught Hospital's supply chains:

Lioba: How did you try to make your work sustainable?

Miki: We tried to work with the hospital management and the supply [centre], so [for] like soap and gloves and just simple basic things like that [...] the hospital would get supplies from like a national [centre], it is part of the government, and they would disperse medications [...].

The process that Miki describes here differs from the supply chains that purpose-built ETCs relied on. Cormack, who worked in a newly constructed, purpose-built treatment centre stated: 'When I was there at [ETC], everything all the stuff was there supplied by the UK government, everything. Most of the medicines, generators, the staff cards all paid for by the UK government.' Miki's description of Connaught Hospital's supply chain, together with Alex's description of materials and conditions in the hospital's EHU, indicates the reality of care work in Sierra Leonean hospitals as not working 'as perfect[ly] as you would want'. The reality of shared risk in Connaught Hospital materialised in low-quality vials and momentary unavailability of correctly mixed chlorine concentrations. For Alex, the decision to take on these added risks and work in a makeshift environment was a political one. They finished the description of their near-exposure as follows:

It was ideologically feeling like this [working in a pre-existing unit] is definitely the best way to do [it], to respond without a doubt, I didn't support the model that a lot of other NGOs were engaging in [temporary purpose-built facilities] for all kinds of reasons but also at the very same time, what felt to me like the additional personal risk was also not nothing. I mean when it happened, when stuff went wrong everybody stuck together and it was a fantastic team […]

Alex closes the analysis of their near-exposure and links their acceptance of shared risk to the environment in which they chose to work and care for Ebola patients. They also justify their decision by clearly opposing the less risky model of working in a purpose-built facility. Here, as in Sharpe (2016), shared risk or, as Alex put it, 'additional personal risk' becomes a political act of caring for Black African life in the wake of colonialism. Rather than adopting an individualised understanding of care, Alex took the global politics that shaped how care could be dispensed during the 2014–16 response in Sierra Leone into account. Such an understanding speaks to the global postcolonial interconnections of care and responsibility (Raghuram et al., 2009). Alex stated: '[The experience] certainly made me think about global health and like neo-colonial agendas of global health in a very different way to how I had before, even though that was always a big question for me […].'

In Alex's account, awareness of neo-colonialism and its implications for global health shape their care practice and influence their theorisation and acceptance of shared risks. For them, shared risk was a political decision, which largely depended on the organisation and infrastructure available in Connaught Hospital. Here, I offer their account as one possible kind of care; an answer to Sharpe's (2016, p. 35) question on how to care for 'lives consigned to the possibility of always-imminent death' in the midst of the Sierra Leonean Ebola epidemic.

Conclusion

In this chapter I have tried to insert care thinking and practice into an analysis of the 2014–16 Ebola epidemic in Sierra Leone. Understanding care, both epistemically and ontologically, beyond its institutional forms allows for a deeper understanding of its historical (and contemporary) conflation with antiblackness, anti-Indigeneity, heteronormativity and ableism. Once we know care by these histories, analyses of its biomedical manifestations in times of humanitarian crisis become, and need to be, complicated. Care in the wake needs to include an awareness of its historical entanglement with antiblackness and of the hold experiences of this conflation had on care recipients in postcolonial Sierra Leone during the epidemic. Care, and differential understandings of care, are also deeply tied to how the human has been conceptualised and to how Black people have long been excluded from this conceptualisation (Wynter, 2001, 2003). In the case of Sierra Leone, the spatial regulations of IPC protocols further (re)inscribed Blackness along an ontological hierarchy, which places Black people at the bottom. In doing so, IPC practices reinforced colonial-racial dynamics of placing Black life ever more firmly in the realm of always-imminent death. On the other hand, care as shared risk can counter the continued violence of the colonial wake. In order to interrupt (post)colonial dependencies, care practices during the Ebola response needed to go beyond traditional biomedical care, such as dispensing medicine, cleaning and feeding patients, to include a political awareness of the entanglement of care and violence and the spatial reproduction of the possibility of death as immanent to Blackness.

4

Wakefulness: Epistemic Spaces, Flows and Epigrammatic Antiblackness

Introduction

In this chapter I take a step back. On the one hand I continue my analysis of global health and antiblackness by focusing on the politics and performance of knowledge during the epidemic response, on the other hand I interrogate the very same politics in relation to my research. Specifically, I analyse the production and circulation of expertise in relation to global health, the Ebola epidemic and antiblackness. I focus on expertise in order to foreground embodied epistemic hierarchies and spatial processes of knowledge production and exchange. Katherine McKittrick (2021, p. 107) asks us to adopt a 'a black sense of place [as] a methodology and an analytical frame that believes in and believes black humanity'. She continues:

> So I ask: What does a black sense of place do to algorithms that presume, in advance, black premature death? How might we shift our methodological questions so that we do not end up in an analytical bind that affirms rather than undoes racial violence?

This chapter points to global health as such an algorithm and tells stories of this analytical bind and how it structured the EVD response and subsequent analyses thereof as well as my research. The epistemic hierarchies and spatial processes of knowledge production described in this chapter reproduce and marginalise antiblackness in global health and, by working to render it invisible, normalise Black African premature death, vulnerability and dependency ever more deeply in existing epistemic and humanitarian structures. The chapter deals with experts, here defined as producers and/or recipients of academic knowledge, and discusses how expertise coincided with colonial-racial hierarchies and constitutes 'an algorithm that presumes, in advance, black premature death' (McKittrick, 2021, p. 107). I argue that both experts and the aforementioned hierarchies influenced the Ebola response but also attend to the partial disruption of colonial continuities by members of the Sierra Leonean diaspora. These disruptions, like the ones detailed in chapter 2, speak to Black African life outside the parameters of antiblackness and white supremacy.

Here I treat expertise as relative specialisation and authority in global health knowledge and practice. As such I oppose it to what Paul Richards (2016) has termed a 'people's science', that is to say local, bottom-up knowledges and approaches to ending the Ebola epidemic. In my analysis I also treat expertise as geographically tethered to white European knowledge production. This is not to say that I consider Europe as the origin of modern knowledge production or indeed 'European knowledge', if it can be so geographically distinct, as universal. Rather I show that white European experts, the knowledge they contributed, and institutions located in Europe and North America, came to play an important role during the British-led response to the Sierra Leonean Ebola epidemic and continue to embody global health expertise. In doing so I also draw on Chanda Prescod-Weinstein's (2020, p. 421) concept of *white empiricism* which stipulates that 'whiteness powerfully shapes the predominant arbiters of who is a valid observer of physical and social phenomena'. Using the example of physics, Prescod-Weinstein shows that the predominance of white men in the professional community produces a double standard in which they fail to apply scientific standards to themselves, while at the same time using those very standards to keep Black women from entering the profession. In this sense, white empiricism ties in with Wynter's writings on the social production of natural sciences. Prescod-Weinstein (2020, p. 422) writes that white empiricism is 'a form of antiempiricism masquerading as an empirical approach to the natural world'. Here, I argue similarly that what counted as expertise or what rendered someone an expert were closely tied to embodied whiteness and to the exclusion of Black experiences from global health. I take expertise to be 'a matter of socialisation into the practices of an expert group' (Collins and Evans, 2008, p. 3). However, while I attend to groups of British-based scholarly experts, healthcare workers and members of the Sierra Leonean diaspora, I take epistemic spaces and flows to be of the utmost importance in my analysis of epistemic politics during and in relation to the Ebola epidemic in Sierra Leone. As I show in this chapter, these point to the simultaneous entanglement and marginalisation of antiblack processes and effects during the response and in its aftermath, and reify Europe as epistemic centre. In this chapter I attend to knowledge on global health and antiblackness both in its studied and personally experienced form. As such I follow Caroline Bressey's (2014, p. 103) invitation to 'put before readers what might be considered more personal aspects of our research practice'.

As in preceding chapters, I show the accumulation of marginalisations of Black life and historical antiblackness that underlay the British-led Ebola response in Sierra Leone, which contribute to normalising Black death, ill health and dependency. I also show how antiblackness manifested itself to me, a Black researcher of global health and geography in my own process of becoming an expert, that is, of conducting academic research, in a space of epistemic production. Overall, I show, following Adia Benton (2016b, p. 270), that in the case of the international Ebola response, the realities of antiblackness and of the colonial wake were 'epigrammatic', that is to say 'situated in a space peripheral or marginal to the main text, hovering over it in ways that make it easy to deny its centrality and significance'. In doing so I extend her work on race and humanitarianism by focusing on colonial continuities.

Apart from Benton's (2016a, 2016b) work on race and humanitarianism, which illuminates the interconnection between whiteness and expertise, I also draw on work on archives by Caroline Bressey (2006) and Marisa J. Fuentes (2018) as well as using Katherine McKittrick's writings to frame my thinking in this chapter. All three highlight the methodological efforts required to unearth Black lives from archives designed to erase them. Yet, as in previous chapters I draw attention to the specifically colonial manifestations of the wake. In doing so I follow Joseph Morgan Hodge's (2007, p. 9) argument that: 'In many ways then, late British colonial imperialism was an imperialism of science and knowledge, under which academic and scientific expertise rose to positions of unparalleled triumph and authority.' Building on his argument, I maintain here that in light of the historical role scientific experts and practitioners have played in the establishment and maintenance of colonial rule, something I have begun to explore in the chapter on mobilities, the epistemic marginalisation of that colonial past by present-day experts warrants close attention. Today, Britain's epistemic power vis-à-vis formerly colonised countries manifests itself by sidelining and ignoring the colonial experience (and the antiblackness that characterised it), rather than dominating it.

Epistemic Spaces

Here I attend to epistemic spaces. Specifically, I analyse two different kinds of spaces that actively contribute to producing and shaping knowledge on the colonial wake and the Ebola epidemic. I analyse awareness of the colonial wake and antiblackness among global health experts. 'Experts' here signifies both the producers and guardians of specialised knowledge. In my analysis of global health and antiblackness, spaces and their location and set-up play an important role in regulating access and conveying epistemic authority. The spaces I analyse here are promoted as producing and guarding knowledge and as prestigious places of scientific innovation. In the first section, I analyse an event that took place at the Royal Society in London, which according to its website is 'a Fellowship of many of the world's most eminent scientists and is the oldest scientific academy in continuous existence' (Royal Society, 2019). In the second section, I relay an autoethnographic account of a racist event that took place in the archives of an international health organisation, where I was conducting archival research. This private organisation is one of the major funders, producers and collectors of medical and health-related knowledge. In this section I draw on (auto)ethnographic accounts of conducting archival research to analyse how global health knowledge and antiblackness coexist in epistemic spaces, yet how the latter remains largely epigrammatic (Benton, 2016b, p. 270).

Expertise and the Marginalisation of the Colonial Wake

The epigrammatic treatment of colonialism in the panel discussion I analyse below signals the colonial wake and the marginalisation of the knowledge that antiblack dimensions of Britain's colonial past in Sierra Leone exist. This encounter reveals how contemporary European epistemic power is manifested by sidelining, rather than dominating, the colonial experience.

In November 2015 I attended a meeting on the global Ebola response in West Africa taking place at the Royal Society in London. The event invitation specified that this was an interactive expert panel discussion presenting the findings and recommendations of an independent panel convened by the London School of Hygiene and Tropical Medicine (LSHTM) and Harvard University, two major academic institutions in the field of global health and tropical medicine. The event was hosted by

Chatham House and the report they were presenting was published in *The Lancet*. In terms of institutional set-up, this event reflected the predominance of British-American expertise and epistemic production in the field of global health. In order to attend the event, I had to register online, provide personal details and an institutional affiliation, and await confirmation of my registration. At the venue, I had to sign in and was issued with a name tag and folder containing relevant information.

In a small room at the Royal Society, about forty people were listening to a series of global health experts, some academic, some professional, some European or American, a few West African, talking about the organisation, development and failures of the global response to the Ebola epidemic. The panellists expert status derived from their seniority in the field of global health, their experience and the institutions they represented.

While some people of colour (mostly West African) spoke, the majority of panellists were white British and North American, as was the majority of the audience. The spatial and racial set-up is noteworthy for several reasons. First, the fact that the event took place in a small room in London, rather than one of the West African countries affected by the Ebola outbreak. This reinforced a dynamic in which the countries in which the epidemic took place were a geographical and political 'borderland' (Duffield, 2001, p. 309), 'an imagined geographical space' governable from a distance and in which the international (health) community could – and felt compelled to – intervene due to the conditions prevailing there. Playing out in West Africa, and predominantly affecting people of African descent, the response was nevertheless thought of and analysed in Britain, by a small handful of (predominantly white) British and American experts. Global health, then, is built on a system, or algorithm in which the expertise deemed necessary to manage Ebola virus disease (and other 'tropical' infectious diseases) resides outside of West Africa, in this case, the UK, and is predominantly accessible to a British, not West African public.

The exchange I focus on here occurred in the second part of the meeting, entitled 'How to rebuild trust in the global system, including the World Health Organization?' This panel consisted of the editor of a medical journal and a professor of global health governance who was also a member of the independent panel. It was moderated by the health editor of a major British newspaper.[1] The moment I analyse here occurred during the Q&A, when a member of the audience asked a question. Because the transcript of the exchange is quite long, I have divided it into segments, which I analyse in turn.[2] Here I trace the marginalisation of colonialism in the Ebola response in panellists' words and their demeanour. The exchange started as follows:

> *Member of the audience*: When the outside world became seriously engaged in this West African outbreak of Ebola, the USA helped Liberia, France went into Guinea and the British went to Sierra Leone. Do you think this neo-colonial division of responsibility is helpful or harmful?

> *Moderator*: [chuckles] That's fascinating. So, who wants to talk about neo-colonialism? [panellists laugh]

> *Editor*: [laughing] Oh God!

> *Moderator*: [turns to Professor] [Professor], do you dare? [laughs; everyone laughs]

> *Professor*: [laughing] Maybe I'll start with the other question [laughs] give [Editor] some time to think about ... [laughs, everyone laughs] [proceeds to answer another question that was asked by someone in the audience on institutional trust]

> [turns to the editor] So [Editor] on the ... [implied: matter of colonialism] [laughs]

The question and the initial reaction to the question, laughter and discomfort, as well as a sense of being overwhelmed ('Oh God'; 'do you dare?') distance the panel members – and the audience more generally – from the topic of (neo-)colonialism. The tone in which the question was asked is earnest, as was the tone of the panel discussion and the questions asked beforehand. The reaction – laughter – seems inadequate and out of touch; the general atmosphere is awkward, given that the question was asked seriously. As Massumi (2015, pp. 8–9) writes, laughter is an 'irruption[s] of something that doesn't fit'. In this situation at the Royal Society however, although the laughter disrupts an otherwise serious discussion of the Ebola response, it seems to work in the opposite way: it counteracts that which does not fit – a question about neo-colonialism – and offers the panellists a vehicle for masking their discomfort, and potentially their fear of having to answer a polarising question. As Delph-Janiurek (2001, p. 417) writes: '"Nervous" laughter can mark sensitive points in conversations at which a potential "danger" has been recognized. This may be a threat to the progression of unproblematic interaction, such as behaviour that somehow threatens the identity or role enacted by one or more inter-actants, disrupting the interactional frame.'

Here, the laughter shifts the terms of the question and the conversation which must follow, back onto a plane that is manageable for the experts on the panel. The question itself did not contest the neo-colonial nature of the international response; it asked if this characteristic was helpful or harmful. The question in itself was not new or unanswered. Sreeram Chaulia (2014), for example, has pointed to the imperial continuity with which former colonial powers intervened in the three countries affected, countries in which they often still hold considerable economic stakes and over which they 'feel a sense of entitlement and privilege' (Chaulia, 2014, n.p.). As Bernadette O'Hare (2015) has pointed out, in *The Lancet*, the Ebola epidemic was exacerbated by structurally underfunded health care systems. This, she argues was partially also due to tax exemptions given to British firms operating in Sierra Leone. According to estimates, between 2014 and 2016 the Sierra Leonean government lost an estimated US \$131 million in tax incentives to firms in the mining and agricultural business (Curtis, 2014). The vast majority of these losses are attributable to tax incentives granted to two London-based mining companies, African Minerals and London Mining. An agreement between the government of Sierra Leone and London Mining prior to 2013, for instance saw a reduction in the statutory income tax from 30 per cent to 6 per cent (Curtis, 2014). The consequences and implications of Britain's continued economic and political influence in Sierra Leone should not have been something to laugh at on a panel debating the international Ebola response.

There is ample literature on humour and laughter as subversive ways of managing colonial, racial or political violence, and as a tool to counter hegemonic structures, such as racism, sexism or neoliberalism (see for instance Casey, 2014; Antoine, 2016; van Roekel, 2016; Pauwels, 2021). In this case the laughter has the opposite effect, however. It does not work against colonial power structures but supports them by, to paraphrase Meghan Corella (2018, p. 120), 'closing off opportunities to interrogate colonial ideologies'. What occurred here was what Corella terms 'white laughter', laughter which constructs public spaces as white, by working towards white innocence while marking critiques of colour-blindness and 'postracialism' by people of colour as disruption. Rather than dealing with the question in earnest, this affective strategy distances the speakers emotionally from both question and topic without having to address their own discomfort and the colonial complicity of the UK, France and the US.

The epistemic space in which the discussion took place was one of critical interrogation around the technical aspects of the epidemic response and of global health governance, which was in no way prepared for discussions of colonial complicity. The question introduces the possibility of such complexity into the room. The moderator's laughter – and both panellists following suit – frames the eventual response to and discussion of the question. Their reaction also masks a potential lack of expertise and delays anyone having to address the question.

The experts on the panel and the moderator delay answering the question for as long as possible. The professor, a woman of colour, does not answer it at all. She directs it to the editor. The exchange continues as follows:

> *Editor*: Oh my God [Moderator laughs]. So just on the, dodging the last question a bit [he proceeds to answer the same question the professor answered]. Now on the neo-colonialism. Ahm boy [audience laughs], I mean it's certainly true that the system as run in global health today retains a lot of features of the colonial system. But that said you know [pauses] I think the countries that went in were trying, I certainly know this from the UK's point of view, I can't speak for the other two [countries], went in to create effective partnerships and if that was driven by history [shrugs] you know let's be careful not to condemn the present because of the sins of the past. I think that we did go into Sierra Leone with the best of intentions – sorry [turns to a member of the audience]?

> *Member of the audience*: It really worked!

> *Editor*: Yeah, yeah and so I prefer to believe that those relationships we have in countries are terribly, terribly important and need to be strengthened.

Again, the editor delays having to answer the last question by concentrating on the question previously already answered by the professor of global health. Here the question of neo-colonialism is pushed aside in favour of another question on institutional trust. He admits to doing so when he says 'again dodging the last question a bit', which expresses feelings of avoidance and discomfort. No one on the panel wants to answer the question, which they shorten to 'neo-colonialism', a move, which strips the question of the complexity with which it was asked. The editor's answer does not state 'Neo-colonialism, in the case of the UK's intervention in Sierra Leone, was helpful', although this is the message that his response conveys. Rather the answer shifts to intentions and motivations and, importantly, separates the past from the present. The editor, is aware of colonialism's problematic nature, referring to it as 'the sins of the past'. These sins, however are moved aside, the colonial past is shrugged off to make way for 'effective partnerships'. Lastly, his admission that he 'prefer[s] to believe' that existing relationships between former colonial powers and West African countries need to be strengthened and are 'terribly, terribly important' again indicates a choice: the violence of the colonial past and its enduring hold can be taken seriously or they can be relegated to the epistemic margins. This relegation reaffirms African and Black dependence on former colonial powers without speaking truth to power, that is to say, without moving beyond the analytical bind which reproduces racial-colonial violence and would complicate this global health story beyond a simple binary of white saviours and Black dependants, and of a nurturing colonial aftermath.

The remark from the back of the audience that 'it really worked' is both pragmatic and outcome-oriented. It does not question whether neo-colonialism was a factor in the outcome of the response. Here the outcome overrides the process and the neo-colonialism that the audience member asked about. Global health is, given the setting in which this conversation took place and due to the nature of its work, outcome-oriented. Global health management is largely taught this way too, to come up with clear, implementable findings that will save human lives.[3] As such, global health and medical experts, as were present during this panel discussion, measured the helpfulness or harmfulness of the neo-colonial nature of the global response in whether or not the epidemic – and the death toll associated with it – could be brought to an end. In this discussion, pre-existing colonial relations allowed a swift deployment of the British-led response. The conversation continued with a remark from the moderator:

Moderator: In fact there is public buy-in too, isn't there? That's the other factor, actually the British are more likely to support Sierra Leone because we had a role there once, I guess.

Member of the audience [nods]: and being francophone or anglophone helped. [...]

[The moderator wants to move on, but another member of audience cuts in]

[*Other member of the audience*]: Look, the Americans at the beginning of September said 'We really want to help Liberia', which was never an American colony, so you can't describe that as neo-colonialism. And President Obama contacted President Johnson-Sirleaf and said 'What do you want?' She said what she wanted, the Americans responded. They said to us 'We have to work inside a multilateral envelope, we created the biggest health mission we've ever done, we've never done one before.' The British came along very quickly afterwards, particularly Philip Hammond and together with the prime minister said, 'We have to help Sierra Leone.' The French came in after that with Guinea. Again, very strong. Thank goodness! Supposing this had been in countries that did not have godparents like these, who just take these amazing decisions. (LSHTM, 2017)

When the other member of the audience speaks, the camera pivots to the audience, where he stands, rather than remain focused on the panellists, which we were able to see before. Some members of the audience nod vigorously throughout his statement. The member of the audience who asked the question smiles and listens intently to his fellow audience member. The mood is one of quiet acquiescence; no one asks a follow up question or visibly disagrees. This might have something to do with the setting in which this event takes place and the format of the discussion, or with the fact that the initial reaction to the question was laughter. The experts are sitting at the front of the room and the audience, many of whom identify themselves as having worked on the Ebola epidemic themselves (they may be considered experts in their own right) are invited to ask questions. The time for questions is limited, however, and throughout this exchange the moderator keeps reminding people to be quick in their contributions and answers.

By responding with a chuckle and an amused 'that's fascinating' the moderator sets the tone in which the question is answered. Her statement about 'British buy-in', is telling. She does not specify the nature of this buy-in or Britain's 'role', nor does she ask whether colonial nostalgia or guilt played a role in Britain's humanitarian concerns. As a 2014 YouGov poll found, 59 per cent of British people interviewed thought that the empire was 'more something to be proud of' than ashamed (19 per cent) (Dahlgreen, 2014). A more recent 2019 poll found that 32 per cent of Britons were proud of the empire, with 27 per cent wanting Britain to still have an empire (Booth, 2020). As such, 'public buy-in' in foreign global health interventions ought to be critically examined. As alluded to in chapter 2, a significant motivation for Britain (and other countries) to get involved in the response was also the fear that Ebola could spread to the UK.

Finally, Liberia. While it is technically true that Liberia was never an American colony, this statement obscures two things. First, Liberia was founded by the American Colonization Society (ACS) in order to remove freed slaves and free African-Americans to territories in Africa. The founding idea of the ACS was that Black Americans would have better chances at freedom on the African continent, rather than in the US; the organisation was tinged with racist ideas around a white America and partially expressed the explicit interests of slave holders (Seeley, 2016; Mbembe, 2017). Lands for colonisation in Liberia were in part procured at gunpoint (Seeley, 2016). As such, stating that Liberia was never an American colony obfuscates the real entanglements between enslavement, the resettlements of freed slaves antiblackness and African colonisation. Such a statement also limits the identity of colonisers to white settlers and administrators. Black colonisation often operated along the same lines as white colonisation. As the history of Liberia and Sierra Leone in the years following the creation of the initial settlements shows, in both societies Black settlers established hierarchies typical of white colonial societies, placing themselves at the top (Kandeh, 1992; Shaw, 2002). Second, this statement adopts a very narrow definition of colonialism as the political and administrative authority over an overseas nation or territory. Such an interpretation negates the wake in that it limits the social, epistemic and psychological effects of colonialism as explored, for instance, by Fanon (2011) or members of the modernity/coloniality group. It also ignores (or chooses to ignore) colonialism's afterlife and the spatial and political dynamics that continue to shape British–Sierra Leonean relations.

Overall, the answers increasingly distance the experts from the premise of the question. Neo-colonialism is only acknowledged – before being repudiated – at the very beginning by the editor, when he starts to answer the question asked by the member of the audience. The negative long-term effects of colonialism are never acknowledged. From then on, all answers explain how Sierra Leone's colonial past was helpful in the organisation of the response. The word 'neo-colonialism' is mostly dropped. The last statement 'Thank goodness. Supposing this had happened in countries that did not have godparents like these' is particularly disturbing. It obscures the violence and exploitation that have characterised British colonial relations with the countries that were forcibly made part of the British empire. At the same time, such a statement implies that countries without colonial *godparents* would be left to themselves, a twist on the Euro-American 'duty to intervene' (Calhoun, 2010) characteristic of the hegemonic nature of humanitarian interventions outside the global North in past decades. In this (post)colonial storytelling, African Blackness manifests as dependence, and the colonial relation, violent though it may have been, as a necessary condition for assisting African countries in the present. The second member of the audience's statement also obscures the history of colonialism, which often is at least partially to blame for the structural deficiencies (Rodney, 1981) that made the Ebola epidemic worse and the local and international responses more difficult.

By attending to the spoken and unspoken reactions of a handful of British-based global health experts, the reality of the colonial present, in the form of a question on neo-colonialism, was both discursively marginalised and not addressed seriously. Contrary to Black Studies' focus on the ability of the past to shape the present, which emphasises historical continuities of antiblackness, 'neo-colonialism' presupposes an old form of colonialism, a rupture and colonial discontinuity. This has repercussions on how global health is taught and how emergency and humanitarian interventions are conceived. The casual treatment of the colonial past and the 'neo-colonial' implications this past brings with it are epigrammatic (Benton, 2016b). The marginalisation and sidelining of past colonial experiences are worrisome tendencies among experts in charge of managing global health in the postcolonial world. The editor's and second member of the audience's statements, and the general way in which the discussion around neo-colonialism is conducted, further contribute to the marginalisation of non-Western experiences of antiblack violence and underscore the reasons why they should be considered in contemporary international disease management. I also want to draw attention to the spatiality of this event. Hosted at and by some of London's most influential scientific institutions, the unchallenged epistemic and discursive marginalisation of the colonial reality by some of the UK's leading global health experts, far from the populations most affected by the epidemic, signals their refusal to acknowledge the reality of the colonial wake as the setting in which the Ebola epidemic and response played out. It also signals their refusal to acknowledge the role European experts play in perpetuating colonial epistemic dependencies between West Africa, Europe and North America today. In the following section I pursue my analysis of epistemic spaces and the interplay of global health knowledge and antiblackness.

Archives and Antiblackness

In this second section I draw on an autoethnography of conducting research on colonial infectious disease control in Sierra Leone at the archive of an international health organisation. The archive in question is a place of historical and medical expertise due to the originality of materials in storage, their historical value and the steps one must take to access this knowledge. As in the previous section, access, and the restriction thereof, becomes an important marker of expertise. Apart from being present in archival materials (texts, documents, photographs), the archival space, its layout and regulations, can itself become a space in which antiblackness is enabled. As Caroline Bressey (2006) has pointed out, Blackness is difficult to trace in archival materials, and at times invisible; tracking it requires attention and care. Marisa J. Fuentes (2018) similarly argues that archives work to silence and erase Black agency, especially that of Black women. While this was also true in the archival materials I studied, I point here to a different experience of 'silencing' both Black women and antiblackness in an archival space.

The Mayor's Commission on African and Asian Heritage 'Delivering shared heritage' report (Barrow et al., 2005, p. 23) called on archives (among other epistemic bodies) to be 'equally accountable to ensuring greater inclusion of African and Asian practitioners'. Since then other writers and historians have described the experience of conducting archival research 'while Black', of feeling out of place and being encountered with surprise and at times being subjected to increased surveillance (Robinson, 2017; Farmer, 2018). The experience I narrate here demonstrates that antiblackness is casually enacted in archives of global health. Its enactment contributes to further silencing Black women in archives, those doing research and those represented or silenced in texts. This enactment also signals an inability to responsibly deal with the colonial and antiblack content contained in archival collections of health and medicine.

In *Dear Science and Other Stories*, Katherine McKittrick (2021, p. 105) writes:

I explore how archives document and institutionalise sexist and racist practices. I argue that because the archives primarily document instances of violence toward and the death of black enslaved people, racism acts as an eerie origin story that can steer us, analytically, toward death. What the archive tells us is what we already know and what we resist, but it can also structure and frame how we enter into the present and future in our writing. [...] If the archive is a knowledge network that records and normalizes black subordination, how do we understand this network outside of itself? What happens to our understanding of black humanity when our analytical frames do not emerge from a broad swathe of numbing racial violence but, instead, from multiple and untracked enunciations of black life?

The following speaks to how archives both 'record and normalise black subordination', not simply in relation to the texts they store but in relation to Black researchers. It also speaks to a researcher's anger and attempts to evade and speak back to archival power, and a refusal to be victimised. Importantly, it showcases how, rather than producing 'objective', that is, white research (Prescod-Weinstein, 2020), for BIPOC, racism is part and parcel of researching health and medicine and this makes neutrality impossible.[4] Neutrality is power, both in terms of doing research unscathed and of not having to speak back or complain. Sara Ahmed (2021, p. 28) describes the 'wear and tear' of coming up against institutions. Working on these paragraphs made for weary experiencing, writing and reading. The story goes something like this:

This is a story of a Black researcher walking into an archive. She fills in all the registration forms and brings the multiple proofs of residence, bank statements, etc. that are required to prove both her identity and that she is not houseless. This takes several trips. Once the registration is complete, she returns to the archive and orders the documents she would like to see. In order to access the room in which the archival material can be seen she needs a reader's pass. This is scanned on an electronic terminal next to the room to grant access (doors open), but also supposedly, to keep track of who is in the room at any given moment. Once in the room she sits at one of a dozen tables.

The layout of the room matters. Not in general, but because of what happens, she remembers. It's not a big room, but it's not small either. It's clean and bright. Some other people work at different tables. Everyone is quiet. To the left of the room from the entrance door is a counter, which gives access to the archives themselves. Only archivists are allowed behind this counter, monitoring what goes on in the room (perhaps), processing requests, fetching documents for the visitors' perusal. The archivists on duty here are not always the same. Sometimes she recognises them from working at the reception counter in the library outside. They seem to be floating between different responsibilities and sections. One woman is particularly nice and friendly. She remembers her fondly.

On this day, she walks up to the counter and hands over her reader's pass. The procedure is the following: Once documents have been ordered, they are processed electronically and (she supposes) ordered files are being fetched and prepared by the archivists on duty. You can only enter the reader's room once your documents have been fetched. So when she walks up to the counter to have her reader's pass scanned, she knows that the documents she's ordered are ready for collection. The archivist on duty is new to her, but for all she knows he's worked here for a long time. This is only her second visit. He hands her the documents she's requested (a few at a time) and she returns to her seat. She peruses. Once finished, she returns the documents to the counter to get her next batch.

Once again, she hands over her reader's pass and once again the archivist scans it into the system to see what to hand over next. This time though, he lingers. On her, on her card and her name. 'Hirsch', he says, 'that's a German name. Why do you have a German name?' She tells him that this is, because she is, in fact, German. 'But your first name does not sound German', he says. She rolls her eyes inwardly and cuts him off. 'It is', she says curtly. 'Where are you from?', he asks and she tells him. Not because it's any of his business, but because she is used to making herself small in front of these questions. Make yourself small, present less of a target and they'll blow over you. But also, because the archive demands it. The organisation's conditions of use tell you that staff will be friendly and respectful. They ask you to be the same. There's no way she will win against this building. She tells him about being Togolese and German. 'Do you speak German?', he asks and she says yes.

He switches to German, which is not his first language, but he speaks it well. This is a small room and the custom is that you speak quietly, so it is unlikely that anyone has been able to follow their conversation up to this point. Now, it is almost guaranteed that they won't be able to. Unless they speak German and have exceptional hearing. He goes to

retrieve her documents and lingers on those too. One of them is marked
with a Colonial Office stamp. 'You study colonialism. Where we try to
help the savages and they throw spears at us,' he says. He laughs. She
forces a laugh. She makes herself small, but also: keeps herself safe. She
does not want an argument with this man. She simply came to look at
old documents. Old documents, which he still holds on to. As well as
her pass. She can't leave this room without her pass. So she stays still.
He tells her about his uncle doing missionary work in Africa. She nods.
'You know', he says, 'the word N***** is not a bad word in my language. It is Latin for Black.' She really wants to leave now, but is frozen
in place. There was nothing in the induction to the archive or archival
rules about what to do in cases like this. No one mentioned that archival
research could entail this. Naively perhaps, she did not prepare herself
for this eventuality.

He still has the documents and her reader's pass. He also needs to
press a button to disable the door and let her out of the room, should
she wish to leave. This is put in place, she assumes, to protect the historical materials available to view here. There are no parameters to protect
her in this place. He tells her a joke about N******. She forces a smile.
Can they become more forced at this point? He asks some more questions about her research then, finally, hands over the documents. She
retreats to her seat, but her seat and the table she is working at are
not far from the counter and he comes over. 'Ms Hirsch', he says, 'I am
sure you will appreciate this joke.' He tells her two more jokes about
N******. Then, shaking with silent laughter he goes back behind the
counter.

She sits in her seat, uncomfortable, averting her gaze. In order to
leave she needs to return the documents to him. At the counter. She
does not want another encounter. So she stays in her seat, even after
she's looked through them all. She stays in her seat until his shift is
over or he's on a bathroom break. Then, when someone else has taken
his place she returns her documents and hastily leaves the room. She
does not go back, but after a few days she writes it all down. She complains via email, but does not hear back. She complains again. This
time about the incident and the delay in acknowledging her complaint.
She hears back eventually and is told that the person working on EDI
[Equality, Diversity and Inclusion] issues is doing so part time and the
inbox wasn't being monitored regularly. They suggest a meeting with
the part-time EDI officer and someone high up in the legal department

to discuss this incident. She wonders if they worry about her going to the press. At the meeting she is told that the person was removed from a customer-facing post. In an email, before or after the meeting, she is not sure, they say that he has been let go. She is not sure what to make of this.

This archival visit becomes a place in which the researcher is subjected to antiblackness in the form of probing questions and racist jokes. While mainly due to the archivist's behaviour, the spatial regulations in place to ensure the safety of rare materials compounded feelings of helplessness and of being silenced. Due to the security-controlled exit of the Rare Materials Room the researcher can't leave without risking being subjected to antiblackness again. The archive and the library that houses it, a place of epistemic production and expertise, had also evidently not trained their archivists in how to interact with non-white visitors and researchers. Nor had they trained them in how to interact with the colonial materials that they have in store. Apart from the many mentions of the N-word, the archivist's reaction to seeing the Colonial Office stamp on one of the documents was inappropriate, although he found it funny. Here again, laughter makes critiques of racism so much harder. Antiblackness manifests itself in this space of health and medical expertise while the spatial regulations (quite typical for archives) left the researcher with little direct recourse to remove herself from the situation without triggering another encounter. Like the Black people in the archives she was researching, she is, in this moment, silenced. Possibly like the Black people in the archives, she silences herself to keep herself safe.

Antiblackness, surfaced not just in the historical and contemporary materials on global health I studied, but also as a result of 'researching while Black' in spaces of epistemic production. The silencing effect of antiblackness experienced here is, I argue, double. First, my silencing increases the accumulation of 'silencings' that Black people in British (and other) historical archives have been subjected to (Bressey, 2006; Fuentes, 2018). Second, the fact that the archivist felt able to display such behaviour is an indication that the historical existence of antiblackness in global health – both in materials and practice – is not considered by places of epistemic production in their effort to shape widely accessible, inclusive places of learning. And there is a third point: laughter (again). As is the case at the Chatham House event, laughter undermines the seriousness of the event. It is not laughter born out of solidarity; it is laughter against

Blackness. As in the case of the moderator, by laughing, the archivist sets the tone for the discussion. Speaking up against the transgression involves now not only contesting the opinion of the archivist, but also the apparent levity of the situation. Laughter in both cases works to disempower the person who takes colonialism, and in this case, racism, seriously.

In the first part of this chapter I have attended to epistemic places. I have analysed two discursive encounters between the production and/or guarding of global health knowledge and expertise and colonialism and antiblackness respectively. The colonial wake, and the awareness of colonial and antiblack violence that it entails, are, I argue, largely marginalised in global health knowledge. The increased encounters with antiblackness that come from being a Black young woman researcher point, however, to the more than epigrammatic presence of antiblackness in places of epistemic global health production. As such, antiblackness and colonialism are epigrammatic, in that they are barely considered by those I encountered during my research, and highly present in that they manifest for researchers of colour. Their epigrammatic nature also repeats the analytical bind, McKittrick (2021) writes about, in that they further the association between African Blackness and dependence or passivity. Furthermore, the spatial regulations of the epistemic places actively made access to both the materials and discussions difficult for the people most affected by antiblackness in global health. The analysis of the international Ebola response took place in London, far away from the populations of Sierra Leone, Guinea and Liberia. This reinforced London's role as epistemic centre and the continuation of colonial power dynamics in which Sierra Leone depends on British expertise. In the second instance, archival spatial regulations, designed to protect historical materials of high epistemic value, made it more difficult to confront the antiblackness I encountered and contributed to the further silencing of Black women.

Epistemic Flows: The Mobilisation of Expertise

In the second part of this chapter I attend to two contrasting types of epistemic flows: the embodied epistemic flows of international, largely white, British-based health responders who travelled to Sierra Leone to work in the Ebola response and the epistemic flows (through communication technologies) that allowed members of the Sierra Leonean diaspora to share relevant knowledge on Ebola prevention with their friends and family in Sierra Leone without travelling there. A big part of the aeromobilities that I discussed in chapter 2 consisted in flying experts from their places of work and residence to the countries in which Ebola was spreading. In other words, aeromobilities were used to connect medical and public health expertise to the places in which it was deemed lacking. In this chapter, I analyse the geographical divide between the places in which expertise 'resides', two of which I have analysed in the previous section, and the places in which, in the case of the Ebola response, it is perceived as missing. I argue that the postcolonial mobility injustice that characterises mobilities between the UK and Sierra Leone shaped the production and embodiment of expertise along colonial and racial lines. These aeromobilities, like the epistemic spaces described previously, contribute to the normalisation of an antiblack reading of Sierra Leone, its inhabitants and, crucially, Black Africans' (in)ability to respond to the epidemic without the intervention of former colonial powers. McKittrick's (2021) analytical bind that repeats racial-colonial violence is present and instrumental in the makings of Euro-American expertise on EVD and the management of the response.

Expertise and Mobility

Sierra Leone's 1913 yellow fever outbreak led to a British infectious disease expert, Rubert Boyce, being sent from London. Like the 1913 outbreak, the 2014–16 Ebola response necessitated the mobilisation of British health experts and practitioners towards Sierra Leone. The conflation of expertise with whiteness was, in the case of the international Ebola response, reinforced through unequal mobility regulations. Here I draw on interviews with international responders to the Ebola response and online materials. I show how colonialism and the antiblack effects of the contemporary mobility regime that enables the marginalisation of Black expertise remain largely epigrammatic in conversations with medical responders to the 2014–16 Ebola epidemic. Building on the previous sections, the wake here manifests in the continuation of Sierra Leone's epistemic dependence on the UK.

Adia Benton (2016b, p. 268) describes how whiteness, in humanitarian interventions, is a placeholder for 'expertise, intellectual capacity, and bureaucratic efficiency and rationality'. As Yuka Suzuki (2018) has exemplified using the case of white Zimbabwean farmers' 'claims of technocratic expertise', this conflation builds in part on racially exclusionary education policies that barred Black Zimbabweans access to education. In colonial Sierra Leone, Black Sierra Leonean access to medical careers was, as I described in chapter 1, in part prohibited (Johnson, 2010). My intention here is not to establish a causal link between the colonial exclusion of Black Sierra Leoneans from obtaining medical expertise and the need for white medical expertise during the Ebola response, but rather to point to the long history of the exclusion of Black Sierra Leoneans from becoming medical experts and the concomitant conflation between whiteness and (medical) expertise in colonial Africa.

In the UK, the NHS, the Department of Health and Public Health England (PHE) put out a call to healthcare workers to volunteer by supporting the UK's Ebola response on 19 September 2014 (Davies et al., 2014). NGOs and bodies had in some instances issued calls for volunteers independently. However, which health experts and practitioners could volunteer for the response depended heavily on repatriation and visa policies. In the recruitment process, the antiblack effects of the regulation of mobilities became visible. Ria, the Ebola response administrator at a medical NGO which sent volunteers to work in Sierra Leone, oversaw the organisation's cooperation and compliance with both DFID (Department for International Development) and PHE, managed volunteers and staff in Sierra Leone, and oversaw their return to the UK.[5] She spoke about the politics of mobility and expertise that came into play in the organisation's recruitment of international volunteers:

> Actually, privileged people got to go, special people. It was like clinicians or like epidemiologists that were like quite famous and excited by Ebola. They were like [sounds excited]: 'Oh my God this is the new thing since HIV and AIDS!' It was really interesting because it kind of showed me the division. There was people applying who had experience in Ebola that were from DRC [Democratic Republic of the Congo], Sudan, Kenya, Uganda that previously worked on other outbreaks but we couldn't recruit them because of repatriation.

Ria's statement alludes to several things. First, the prestige associated with working on the Ebola response by career clinicians. According to her statement, some clinicians interpreted Ebola as an event furthering their expertise on infectious disease control, outbreak management or tropical diseases. Second, she alludes to the visa politics that shaped the organisation of the response, which meant that some health workers and medical experts who had experience of working on haemorrhagic fevers could not deploy to Sierra Leone because it was not certain whether their countries of origin would take them back. While Ria speaks of African citizens, I draw attention to the underlying Blackness, which has long regulated Sierra Leoneans' international mobility. She continued by explaining:

> At the time that the Ebola outbreak happened there was only some countries that would repatriate their citizens if they had Ebola. So certain countries wouldn't repatriate their citizens and certain countries would. So for example America, Canada and most of Europe would whereas some of the other countries would not. Let's say we recruited someone from DRC, if they got Ebola we couldn't send them back to their home country so therefore we couldn't recruit them.

Here Ria attests to the differential mobility potential of health experts and practitioners who wanted to volunteer in the Ebola response. In both statements Ria opposes European and North American countries like the UK or Canada to African countries, like the DRC, Sudan or Uganda. Two things contributed to differential mobilities during the Ebola epidemic: the first being health infrastructures in experts' countries of origin. Fearing their inability to contain potential outbreaks of their own, many African countries refused to repatriate health care workers who volunteered in the Ebola response. Second, and relatedly, health care workers from these countries could not be repatriated to the UK, even if they volunteered for a British organisation, such as the one Ria worked for. Anton, who worked for the same organisation alluded to this when he explained that medevacs were not going to be made available for all nationalities of volunteers. I have quoted him more extensively on this in chapter 2, but part of his statement is worth repeating. He confirmed Ria's statement by saying that 'I think we did not take volunteers from other African countries because we didn't know what would happen if they got sick.'

Alex explained their personal experience with this:

> When we had that conversation if I needed to be evacuated, they said I would have the choice: UK or SA [South Africa], but they recommended that I should go to the UK and I – my father is from the UK, so I actually have two passports – and so I quarantined in the UK because SA wouldn't let me come back home afterwards [...]. It was a little bit annoying because I actually had some stuff I needed to do back home [laughs]. I was advised to go to the UK, because someone else had been

sent back from SA and then sent back to Freetown and so I was like, I felt like I might get stuck in this loop.

Alex's quote shows that volunteering one's expertise and experience in the Ebola response was dependent on having a powerful passport, but also that this influenced one's chances of receiving high-quality medical treatment in the case of an infection. Alex, a South African, was able to participate in the response because their British passport allowed them safe repatriation in the case of infection. This possibility was not available to a majority of African health experts and practitioners. Indeed, as Benton (2014) has argued, repatriation regulations were subjected to racial/national differentiation as became clear with the WHO's refusal to provide funds for the repatriation of Sierra Leonean doctor Olivet Buck. In the same week two Dutch healthcare workers were repatriated after coming into contact with the virus (Barbash, 2014; Benton, 2014). The marginalisation of Black expertise takes two forms. On the one hand it consists of restricted mobilities, which made it difficult or impossible for Black African experts to safely participate in the Ebola response. On the other hand, as in the case of Dr Olivet Buck, Black medical expertise and the capacity to care for Sierra Leonean patients infected with Ebola is marginalised, or rather eliminated, through death. Simultaneously this led to an Ebola response in which the conflation between whiteness and expertise was exacerbated.

Ria spoke to this in her interview:

We were sending Sierra Leoneans to the UK to be trained or to conferences across the world to be able to share their experience or upscale people because of the number of healthcare workers that died. So there were definitely positives and negatives. However, because of the lack of mobility of being Sierra Leonean that also sometimes became problematic, like trying to get visas to send someone to Turkey or a Sierra Leonean to South Africa was quite problematic because you had a Sierra Leonean passport, whereas if you have a UK passport I'll most probably be able to blank [reserve] you a space in a UN flight. Like, the privilege that comes with the locality of your passport, changes everything. And that became apparent in the outbreak. Who could be sent, who could not be sent. Which countries we would repatriate [to], which ones [we] wouldn't.

Ria explains a direct link between expertise and mobility injustice. She details that upscaling Sierra Leoneans' knowledge was dependent on the access their passports granted them to various countries. This also meant a decreased ability of Sierra Leoneans to shape global knowledge on EVD and contribute their expertise to the epistemic canon influencing its management. Ria opposed this to the possibilities for humanitarian mobility that came with a UK passport and how this inequality intensified during the Ebola outbreak. Infectious disease control intersected with postcolonial mobility regulations and laid the unequal access to global mobility bare. This unequal access largely operated along colonial-racial lines, making it once again more difficult for Black Sierra Leoneans/Africans to get involved in the response and build their expertise.

At the other end of the spectrum were British medical professionals who volunteered in Freetown. Tom, a clinical doctor, told me how he ended up working there:

> I was then in [region] doing my Master's on [infectious disease] and there were no rains, the [rainy] season did not come in [region] and therefore there were no [vectors] and therefore there was no [infectious disease] and then I saw that there was another viral haemorrhagic fever happening and decided that I'd go. Didn't really know much about what the job would entail, but yeah, I guess felt like I was doing something worthwhile and decided to stay.

Tom's statement alludes to what Ria, the recruitment manager, critiqued about the recruitment process. It is somewhat at odds with the social justice motivations that some other volunteers displayed in statements such as, 'I've never volunteered before, always wanted to' and 'I've always wanted to help people who are less fortunate than us' (Cormack, interview with the author, 2017); and 'I really wanted to go […] I guess that's the symptom of people who want to save the world' (Dina, interview with the author, 2017). Tom chose where to study infectious diseases and where to work, how long to stay and where to intervene in medical emergencies. After finishing work on the Ebola epidemic he took up a more permanent post in Sierra Leone.

The furthering of Tom's expertise and experience was dependent on his ability to move without constraints. He was not the only volunteer whose career had involved travel and experience of working in a medical context in a different country. According to Ria, the NGO she worked for actively recruited people with experience working in 'low-income settings'. Many volunteers thus had previous experience of working in settings outside of the UK. This contributed to their recruitment. Gareth for instance, an infectious diseases doctor, spent two months living and working in Southern Africa while at medical school. Dina, an epidemiologist who worked for a different organisation, had experience of working in Senegal. At the same time this form of expertise, like the clinical expertise of treating haemorrhagic fevers, was at times seen as universally applicable. One responder with previous work experience stated, 'I worked in Malawi for a year. I am familiar [with] what an African town looks like' (Hector, interview with the author, 2017). Such a statement reflects the belief that European knowledge and experience are universally applicable, but also minimises the cultural and political diversity of sub-Saharan Africa. The postcolonial politics of mobility led to a situation in which the association between whiteness and expertise was exacerbated. Though not intentionally racialised, the effects of the regulation of mobilities during the Ebola epidemic coincided with the mobilisation of predominantly white European and North American expertise and a marginalisation of opportunities for Black African involvement and upscaling.

The association of whiteness and expertise that is discussed by Benton (2016b) or Suzuki (2018) intersects with the regulation of postcolonial mobilities during the Ebola epidemic. Though not intentionally racialised, the effects of this regulation nevertheless led to a situation in which Black expertise was marginalised at the same time as white expertise was mobilised. This inequality relied largely on European/North American passports affording their carriers far more mobility – and the reassurance of repatriation – than those of African and especially Sierra Leonean responders. The colonial wake manifested in intensifying Sierra Leone's dependence on the UK (and Europe more generally) in terms of medical expertise and capacity while further marginalising Sierra Leoneans' ability to build up their capacity to contribute to the response.

In the final section I focus on the making of expertise in the colonial wake by considering the efforts of members of the Sierra Leonean diaspora in the UK and Europe to communicate and share knowledge relevant to the response with their friends and families in Sierra Leone.

Making Knowledge in the Wake

The Sierra Leonean diaspora in the UK was actively involved in the British-led Ebola response (Purvis, 2014) and its members became EVD experts in their own right. To underline their epistemic authority, they gave interviews to major news outlets, advised the NHS and RedR (the organisation tasked with preparing NHS volunteers to be sent out to Sierra Leone, RedR, 2010) on cultural norms and provided briefs about dos and don'ts in Sierra Leone more generally. Some members of the diaspora travelled back to Sierra Leone to work in either governmental, non-governmental or international organisations on the ground. As David Rubyan-Ling (2019) has illustrated, big parts of the diaspora were at the onset of the epidemic unaware of the existence and the medical and societal implications of Ebola. Other authors have analysed the diaspora's use of technology (Abdullah, 2017) and, while I touch on the means of communication that were used by the diaspora to communicate with their families and friends back home, I focus on the processes and dynamics that turned members of the Sierra Leonean diaspora into experts. Building on Rubyan-Ling's (2019) work on social remittances and the ascription of expertise and authority to expat Sierra Leoneans, I show that expertise is both relative and relational and that it is tied in with geographical location and postcolonial positionality. At the same time, the diaspora created expertise and this at once relied on and surpassed colonial power structures and colonial epistemic flows. I start by exploring the juncture between expertise and race, the role that it played in the Ebola response and how it was navigated by members of the diaspora. I then focus on localised examples of the creation of Ebola-related expertise by members of the diaspora.

McKittrick (2021) and other Black Studies authors alongside her argue for a reading of Blackness that exceeds death and racist violence, exclusions and marginalisation. Following her lead, I want to examine how the diaspora 'made' expertise in the wake or how they came to be experts in a humanitarian and epistemic environment in which, as I have shown in my discussion of the Ebola panel discussion, Black expertise and the antiblack reality of the colonial present were largely epigrammatic, and in which Blackness was heavily associated with dependence.

Interviews with members of the diaspora illustrated how far expertise correlates with authority and how authority intersects with nationality and race. I have drawn on Benton's (2016b) analysis of the conflation between expertise and whiteness in the previous section, but show here the extent to which this conflation came to play a role in international responders' pre-deployment training.

This racial-epistemic hierarchy became visible when interviewees spoke about the training that British-based healthcare workers attended before being deployed by the NHS. Members of the Sierra Leonean diaspora in the UK were involved in the design and delivery of these training sessions. In the UK, RedR UK, an organisation which 'provides training and technical support to NGOs, aid workers and communities responding to natural and man-made disasters all over the world' (RedR, 2010) was responsible for training NHS healthcare workers for their deployment to Sierra Leone to work in Ebola treatment centres (RedR, n.d. a). Cormack, one of the white British NHS volunteers I interviewed, told me about his experience in these training sessions:

> Before we went out, a week before we went out they said that Sierra Leoneans have a lot of respect for white people and I found that a really strange thing for someone to say, but they told us that a couple of times, even the Sierra Leonean people that came to talk to us about culture and language.

Cormack reacted with bewilderment to this statement. So much so that he felt it necessary to raise it with me when I asked him about the training in our interview. I asked him to elaborate:

> So we were told that a couple of times, I don't know [pauses] white people, British people and I think it's probably a lot to do with the civil war. Or it might not be. But I met people there who wanted Britain to take Sierra Leone back as a British colony. Oh yeah. I don't know, I might have a picture, some of the buildings along the way to Kerry Town [ETC], had Union Jacks painted on them stuff like that, yeah I'm not joking! [...] And people said to me as well 'We need the British back, we need you to come back!' And the thing was, it was a long-term British colony a long, long time ago and [...] freed slaves were settled there and there was a lot of – back in the 1800s – of philanthropy and people set freed slaves up in their own town and all that. [...] But we were actually told on the first week that you know that they look up to British people or white people and I found that really strange. But I don't know. I don't know if I saw that really. Working with Sierra Leoneans I saw that [pauses] I think there was a lot of acknowledgement of our skills, they wanted to learn, but that's not looking up to someone, is it?

Cormack refers to the history of British involvement in Sierra Leone. This, he qualifies as important while also distancing himself from it. His statement shows the tension or unease that can surface when talking about colonialism. He seems to underline the importance of colonialism ('It was a long-term British colony') while at the same time placing it in the distant past, which strips it of some of its importance ('It was a long, long time ago'). He does not make the connection between his knowledge of the colonial history of Sierra Leone and what he was told by Sierra Leoneans during his RedR training about whiteness and authority. His detailed description of the pre-colonial philanthropic era – more detailed than that offered by most of the people I interviewed – was followed by insecurity and hedging 'I don't know if I saw that [respect/deference towards white people] really. [...] that's not looking up to someone, is it?' He also seemed to hesitate over which group – white people or British people or both – he was told was highly respected. While he was aware of Britain's history in Sierra Leone he did not see how colonial continuity could manifest as respect towards whiteness.

I asked members of the Sierra Leonean diaspora who had been involved in contributing to and delivering the training sessions about the sessions too. Isata, a young Sierra Leonean-British woman, who had worked on the presentation used in the training sessions, confirmed that they had included a segment on whiteness and authority in the trainings (Fieldwork notes, 2017). So did Brima, a member of the Sierra Leonean diaspora in the UK. When I asked him whether whiteness was generally associated with authority in Sierra Leone, he stated:

It's unfortunately true [laughs] [...]. When I was at the BBC I was the person making the programme, [but] they [Sierra Leoneans] kept going to my producer to speak to and he had to keep saying 'He's my boss, go and speak to him.' It's one of the things that annoys me that you could send two people to Sierra Leone one black and one white and they'd pay more attention to the white person. [...] So there's – it's really bad in Sierra Leone. I can't stress how bad it is, but that is true, they give a sort of respect and kudos to a white person that they would just not give to a black person that is of equal or higher authority, but it's true, it's unfortunately true.

Brima's statement and the personal example he gave illustrate how, as Benton (2016b) states, whiteness, expertise and authority interact with one another. Brima does not give any background information on the racial and epistemic hierarchy that he sees playing out in Sierra Leone and that he has experienced himself, but he emphasises it at several points ('It's really bad in Sierra Leone. I can't stress how bad it is'). His statement also alludes to the complicated politics of race and authority. In his interpretation, the objective nature of authority is subjected to the reality of being Black and the lack of expertise that is often associated with Blackness.[6] Brima continued his statement about deference towards whiteness by speaking explicitly about how he advised healthcare volunteers who were deploying to Sierra Leone as part of the Ebola response:

> I'd also say to them [trainees] because of that [unquestioned deference towards whiteness] be careful of what you say because you could be talking rubbish and they won't challenge you because you're white. They'd challenge me because I'm black, but they'd let you go ahead talking absolute garbage and not say: 'Hm, sorry but that's not correct.' And so be very careful about what you say, how you say those things because people will be nodding at you and then take you down the wrong alley when they should be saying 'No! Stop and turn back.' And they won't and that's something, as I said it's something that really annoys me. [...] It's a fact of life.

Brima's concluding remark, 'It's a fact of life', is telling about the reality of being Black and working alongside white colleagues in Sierra Leone. Brima cautioned volunteers who participated in the training to think carefully about their whiteness and their expertise. As he states, and this is again in line with Benton's (2016b) analysis, whiteness and expertise are often perceived to go hand in hand in Sierra Leone. This becomes especially clear in his statement that 'you could be talking rubbish and they won't challenge you because you're white'. Cormack confirms Brima's training, unwittingly perhaps, when he states that 'there was a lot of acknowledgement of our skills', although he does not interpret this to be deference or undue authority. As such, the cautioning that Brima expressed, and that Cormack heard did not necessarily translate into the same sense of understanding of expertise and authority. Despite the association of whiteness, authority and expertise that Brima warned trainees about, Cormack, in his interpretation, questions whether the deference he experienced had anything to do with whiteness. Their differential interpretation is linked to their different experiences of the colonial wake. For Brima, a Black British-Sierra Leonean man living and working in the UK, the conflation between whiteness and expertise/authority was a fact that he had experienced in his own life. For Cormack this information was new (and possibly uncomfortable). In comparison to Brima, Cormack was not 'awake' (Sharpe, 2016) to the reality of colonial-racial hierarchies that permeated (and continue to permeate) knowledge in the aftermath of colonialism.

The time of the epidemic and response, however, was also one in which the diaspora was placed in a position of authority with regard to their Ebola-related knowledge. This authority especially played out in relation to the diaspora's communication with friends and family back home. In these instances, the Sierra Leonean diaspora were geographically closer to and seemed to have more authoritative access to Ebola-related knowledge than the Sierra Leoneans they communicated with back home. This was illustrated in an interview with a member of the Sierra Leonean diaspora living in Germany. Solomon had read up on the origins of Ebola in the Congo, how it spread and that there was, in early 2014, no cure. He told me the following:

So I called my village. I told my village – I am the village elder – 'Stay at home. Be careful and have little contact with others. Let them say that you are conservative, but this is how it should be done. Ebola is a disease that is transmitted easily.' [imitates villagers' scepticism] 'Yes, but brother we are safe here.' I said: 'No, no one is safe. No one is safe from Ebola.' (author's translation)

Solomon's quote illustrates the role of expert and advisor that some members of the diaspora took on. Solomon used his authority of being both a village elder and a member of the diaspora living in Germany. In this case, he gave the people in his village in Sierra Leone direct instructions on how to behave. He did not give them any information that they could not have gotten from local officials. Rural African communities have long known how to establish basic protection against infectious diseases, such as smallpox (Richards, 2016; Piot, 2012). However, the fact that Solomon called from Germany to warn them against the Ebola virus added authority to his directive. Here, as in relation to whiteness, expertise and authority are linked to living in Europe. In Solomon's case this authority stretches so far as to be able to contradict and overrule the opinions of the people in his village in Sierra Leone ('Yes, but brother we are safe here' – 'No, no one is safe').

Solomon also used his position to try to transmit the knowledge he had accumulated by speaking to friends and drawing on the sources of information available to him. This involved some form of epistemic translation. He described this to me in the following exchange:

Solomon: I also really tried to explain to them in my language, not in Krio, in the language that they understand. Because the vocabulary differs. But in my language, although there is no name for Ebola [...] we developed a name for it.

Lioba: What is the name?

Solomon: Tumbu. Tumbu means maggot. [...] It looks like a maggot [both laugh]. So we said tumbu and we tried to explain what it means in our language. And you know in our language this tumbu, the maggot can enter people and when that happens, then it can draw out blood. So we tried to speak in this way. And then they understood. It was not fearmongering. It was the reality of what we could transmit in the language's vocabulary. (author's translation)

Here, Solomon translates his knowledge of Ebola into knowledge that has local currency. His translation of EVD into 'tumbu' and his exclamation 'It looks like a maggot' rely on his knowledge of Ebola being a filovirus and his acquaintance with the appearance of the virus under a microscope. He states, 'It was the reality of what we could transmit in the language's vocabulary', a statement which acknowledges both Ebola's microbiological nature as well as the necessities of making the disease intelligible for the people living in his native village. Here expertise becomes a practice of both linguistic and epistemic translation.

Solomon's statement echoed that of another member of the diaspora, Musa, a Sierra Leonean doctor working in London. Musa stated that when communicating with fellow members of the diaspora or with family and friends in Sierra Leone, his emphasis was less on whether or not Ebola was real, but rather that even if it was not real it still had the potential to kill:

You know you would also during those conversations [with family and friends in Sierra Leone] sometimes hear that: 'Oh is this real?' [...] I think there is a difference between, you know, 'Is this real?' and actually 'Do I believe that if I got this it could kill me?' [...] But people who were still certain it [Ebola Virus] was 'man-made' towards the end and whatever their reason for it being 'man-made' whether it had just been imported by other people or whether it was not really a virus, but they still believed 'Ok it may have been man-made but actually if I got it, this time it's real, it can do damage.' So there was that shift there and for me actually that was the more important thing, not whether you think it's man-made or not, but whether you thought this is dangerous and that I should stay away from crowded areas, not go to funerals, etc., all the things that they were advising.

By focusing on the reality of danger rather than the reality of the virus, Musa's attention was less on whether his interlocutors could understand expert microbiological and epidemiological knowledge, and more on how to get them to observe safe practices. His acknowledgement that the deep-seated mistrust towards biomedical explanations of the disease would harm prevention efforts led him to initiate a shift in how he shared knowledge pertaining to Ebola. This effort at epistemic translation is a form of expertise that did not rely on Sierra Leoneans' understanding of Ebola's aetiology, but rather took into account the hoped-for impact. In the wake of colonial medical campaigns and accumulations of distrust (Coultas, 2020), effective Ebola expertise required taking this distrust into account and adjusting the way in which public health advice was communicated. In other words, it required a 'wakefulness' (Sharpe, 2016) to the entanglement of biomedical expertise and colonial and antiblack violence.

Other conversations with members of the diaspora evidenced similar practices, if not of translation, then of communication. They were similarly imbued with authority. Aminata told me how she communicated with her cousins in Sierra Leone:

Like my cousins I was always calling them in Sierra Leone: 'You guys better listen to what they're telling you. Don't go out when they're giving you a curfew.' Because some of them wanted to be going out because they thought 'Oh no it's not …'. I was calling them religiously every single week. Getting my mum to call her sisters to tell them. To say: 'This is what we're hearing. You guys need to stay home! Don't go near this area. This is where it's coming from!' And so even doing that, calling them and telling them and they were saying 'No we know now how serious it is.' I said, 'For now you pray at home, because you shouldn't be in big crowds' and stuff. But they, they listened.

Aminata's tone, when she describes calling her cousins is authoritative. Aminata was not telling her cousins anything that they were not being told in Sierra Leone at the time. In fact, she told her cousins to listen to local authorities ('You guys better listen to what they're telling you. Don't go out when they're giving you a curfew'). She also told them what she was hearing on the news and in the UK. At the end of her statement her cousins, it seems, had understood the seriousness of the situation. Whether this was due to her repetitive calls or due to the development of the epidemic in Sierra Leone or any other factor is unclear, but Aminata's authority is evident in her concluding remark 'they listened'. As in Solomon's case, Aminata's location in Europe imbued her knowledge with authority and made it expertise. This coincides with Rubyan-Ling's (2019) analysis of health expertise as a form of social remittance during the Sierra Leonean Ebola outbreak. Building on his argument, I would however stress the continued colonial implications that these remittances carry in that here, expertise is performed along colonial lines. The authority that in the previous section of this chapter accompanied whiteness is here embodied through a European location and increased access to European information and expertise. Europe is still reified as epistemic centre.

At the same time, due to the diaspora's relative epistemic authority on Sierra Leone in the UK, their involvement in the response also signals a more subversive use of epistemic power. The diaspora's role during the Ebola response, their making of expertise, is an example of transcending discourses on Black Africanness, which condemn Africans to dependence and passivity and which, in so doing, facilitate a grammar of racist violence. On the one hand, their geographical position and the authority that is conferred upon them by people in Sierra Leone reproduce the UK and its residents as a powerful epistemic centre. On the other hand, acknowledgement of the intersection between whiteness and expertise by members of the diaspora, and the active role they took on in training NHS volunteers deployed to Sierra Leone, challenges the traditional epistemic hierarchy between former colony and former coloniser and between Black and white. This challenge is somewhat mitigated by the admission of perceived white epistemic superiority. At the same time, members of the diaspora took it upon themselves to communicate with friends and family in Sierra Leone and to transmit knowledge and concepts that would lead to a reduction in new Ebola infections.

Conclusion

An analysis of epistemic hierarchies shows how McKittrick's (2021) 'analytical bind' shapes and sustains antiblackness in global health. Epistemic hierarchies work along embodied and geographical colonial-racial lines and manifest in epistemic places and flows. This revealed a continuation of Sierra Leone's perceived and produced epistemic dependency on the UK. This is a sign of the colonial wake and the ways in which the Ebola epidemic took place in its midst, yet was not taken into account in high-profile analyses of the response, such as the Ebola response panel at the Royal Society discussed here. There are various ways in which antiblackness and colonialism were treated as epigrammatic (Benton, 2016b) while also manifesting in places of epistemic production. This signals a lack of 'wakefulness' (Sharpe, 2016) to the importance of the colonial wake in global health research and practice. Drawing on work by Bressey (2006) and Fuentes (2018) on the silencing of Black people in historical archives, I have sought to extend their analyses to the physical space of the archive. The unchallenged existence of antiblackness in places of epistemic production echoes the spatial, epistemic and practical entanglements with antiblackness that characterised British medical interventions in Sierra Leone during colonial times.

Focusing on the interplay between mobility and expertise, and attending specifically to the links between postcolonial 'passport privilege' (Ria, interview with the author, 2017), whiteness and the making of expertise further contributes to critical analyses of aeromobilities. A focus on the role of the Sierra Leonean diaspora in the Ebola response shows how race and expertise intersect, and how members of the Sierra Leonean diaspora translated information and knowledge to their families and friends in Sierra Leone. While my analysis in this chapter drew especially on work by Benton (2016b), I try to extend her analysis of race as epigrammatic in humanitarian interventions by taking the colonial wake into account. While the marginalisation of race in humanitarian interventions deserves attention, I have here sought to highlight the convoluted interplay of colonial-racial hierarchies in the production and circulation of global health knowledge, that signals the colonial wake.

5

Thinking Global Health Otherwise

I write this in lieu of a conclusion. It feels difficult to conclude on structures that are ongoing, even after the official end of an event. It's been ten years since the beginning of the West African Ebola outbreak. As I edit this book, global health institutions and governments are failing the people of Gaza. Again. I wanted to resist the urge to draw comparisons to the situations we find ourselves in today: still in the midst of an ongoing pandemic (Covid), whose toll on human lives and the lives of those who do not claim an able-bodied, white, middle-class, cis-gendered bodies in particular, is increasingly being ignored by governments the world over. In the midst of another brutal war on the people of Gaza, of the denial of human dignity and rights. All three: Ebola, Covid-19 and the deliberate attacks on health infrastructures in Gaza and violations of patient and human rights, are singularities. Yet there are commonalities and similarities here too. Let us notice these and build solidarities. Not everything is antiblackness, but everything is linked to supremacist modes of thinking and governing. This ongoing-ness, this repetition, is the reason why this book is entitled *Antiblackness and Global Health* and not *Antiblackness and Ebola*. The structures which shaped one global health event, shape our lives as we move through the next one and the one after.

What this research has taught me are ways of knowing the British-led Ebola response differently; of reading global health otherwise. Hopefully, I have been able to share these ways with you. I want us to understand the wake as a political and geographical reality that affects all of us. I want us to notice, again and again, how antiblackness and colonialism are at once normalised and marginalised in global health and in the Ebola response. I propose that we take colonial infrastructures seriously, and that we pay attention to their endurance and the ways in which they shape global health. A challenge: Let us politicise and interrogate practices of care. Let us approach them with caution. Finally, an invitation: To use care as methodology in global health research and beyond. To live caring and careful lives. To learn, teach and share with care.

Instead of bringing things to a close at this moment, I want to blast them wide open. To think about not what we have learnt, but all the things we are still to (un)learn; to think about thinking global health otherwise. Depending on your outlook on and experience of the world, you may think that that is what I have done in this book. To a certain extent that is correct, but there is room for so much more. We need to go and think much further. To think global health otherwise, to think it beyond and against the antiblack and colonial forces that continue to hold it, requires an act of courage. We need to abandon the structures of how to think the world and enter the unknown. The unknown is a scary place, but for many of us, in health and elsewhere, the known is just as scary.

In *Experiments in Imagining Otherwise*, Black British feminist writer Lola Olufemi (2021, p. 32) writes

> My aim is to produce a map that is nothing like a map at all but rather a record of traces that make connections between the past(present/ future)—the present(future/past)—and the future (past/present). I want to demonstrate how these temporal regimes encroach on one another, so to tell the story of the past means telling the story of the present, which is already where the future resides. Maybe time is a many-pronged spiral: a thick and firm approach and retreat, steady and unrelenting. The place where memory and repetition are disguised and reconfigured.

This book tries to tell the story of the past and the present, which, as Olufemi puts it, 'is already where the future resides'. To think the past as simultaneous to the present and future means taking the legacies we are left with seriously and not underestimating their ability to continuously structure the world we inhabit. Global health's future seems to hang in the balance, except it also seems like it was decided long ago and is being made right now. How do we escape the fatalism of this future/present/ past coincidence? How do we simultaneously abandon temporal linearity and work against the cyclical nature of antiblackness and coloniality that seems to offer little escape? That is the double-edged sword of conceptual antiblackness. It allows us to see and to infer perspectives previously ignored in global health. As I wrote in the introduction, I don't want us to be left with a sense of doom and inescapability. Racism and antiblackness mean that we, and here I mean all of us, white people and Black people and Indigenous people and everyone, already don't have all of the options. 'We live in an anti-Black world – a systemically anti-Black world; and therefore whites are not [simply] "racists". They too live in the same world in which we live. The truth that structures their minds, their "consciousness", structures ours.' Wynter's (2006, n.p.) words still ring true. I want to think global health otherwise, but in order to do this, I need global health to think differently about antiblackness and coloniality. We need to abandon the belief that colonialism is a thing of the past, that antiblackness only exists between certain latitudes and longitudes, that white supremacy is an American invention and that racism on the African continent only manifests in Southern Africa. Most importantly, we need to abandon the idea of health and science as apolitical.

To paraphrase Olufemi (2021, p. 43), we need to redefine the realm of the possible. To courageously imagine what global health could look like if we weren't held by the epistemic constructs of the present. To think beyond the moral imperative to save lives. This, I think, is important and daunting all at once. I propose in this book that Black Studies offers a way out of global health's epistemically and physically oppressive structures, although by no means the only way. Black Studies enables a focus on the structuring and pervasive power of antiblackness and its hold on Black (and white) life in the colonial wake. Black Studies explicitly challenges how we study antiblackness and offers approaches to locating and foregrounding it in silences and the margins to which it has often been relegated. In this book I have used Black Studies to think about how (medical) care and antiblackness have been, and continue to be, entangled in global health. Rather than focusing on individual racism or prejudices, Black Studies adds an important lens to the study of global health interventions, which challenges the (a)political stance of global health and medicine and examines the continuing prevalence of its own colonial and antiblack past. Specifically, this allows for a broadening of perspectives and a re-centring of issues of colonialism and antiblackness in contemporary analyses of global health interventions, both of which were, in my research, largely epigrammatic.

Olufemi begins her book with words I want to borrow to end mine. She writes (2021, p. 17) 'The otherwise requires a commitment to not knowing. Are you ready for that?'

I think we need to learn to be.

List of Interviewees

Interviewees are listed in the order in which they appear in the book.

Pseudonym	Interview date	Interview location
Anton	25/07/2017	London, UK
Dina	22/05/2017	London, UK
Charlotte	24/08/2017	London, UK
Gareth	25/07/2017	Online interview
Alex	04/08/2017	Online interview
Anne	17/08/2017	London, UK
Emmanuel	22/08/2017	Online interview
James	24/08/2017	London, UK
David	06/06/2017	London, UK
Brima	10/07/2017	London, UK
Aminata	31/05/2017	London, UK
Tom	02/08/2017	Online interview
Anika	03/08/2017	London, UK
Maria	14/08/2017	Online interview
Laura	05/10/2017	London, UK
Hector	09/08/2017	Online interview
Jack	22/08/2017	London, UK
Ria	12/06/2017	Online interview
Miki	17/08/2017	London, UK
Cormack	10/07/2017	Phone interview
Solomon	25/06/2017	Berlin, Germany
Musa	01/08/2017	London, UK

Notes

Preface

1. Here I use the concept of the hold to describe how Black life is lived and understood in reference to the antiblack past. The direct impact of this past can, like a hold, be firm or loose. To say that the past 'holds' Black life in the present accounts for this range of grips.

Introduction: Thinking Towards Black Humanity in Global Health

1. The stories that make up these constellations have been reported, in whole or in part and using various points of views, in the media. The most complete tracings of the death of Dr Khan available to me were by Tim O'Dempsey (2017) in the MSF anthology *The Politics of Fear* and subsequently by Sierra Leonean journalist Abdul Rashid Thomas (2019a) for the *Sierra Leonean Telegraph* in July 2019. My retelling of events relies on their work and that of other journalists.

2. I first heard of Dr Olivet Buck's passing when reading Adia Benton's *somatosphere* article 'Race and the Immuno-logics of the Ebola Response in West Africa' (2014).

3. The Decolonising Global Health movement rose to prominence in late 2019/ early 2020, spurred on by various student-led conferences at prominent public health schools in the US and Europe. The movement's aims are to critically interrogate global health's colonial origins and its enduring power dynamics, to challenge the West's hegemony in the field and to empower Black, Indigenous and Communities of Colour.

1 Place, Weather and Disease Control in (Post)Colonial Freetown

1. Interview with Sierra Leonean historian Dr Sylvanus Spencer in Freetown, 30 May 2016.

2. The full inscription on the plaque reads: 'Royal Hospital and Asylum for Africans rescued from slavery by British valour and philanthropy Erected AD MDCCCXVII His Excellency Lieut. Col. MacCarthy, GOV'.

3. For a detailed account of the architectural development of Connaught Hospital, see Koutroumpi (2020).

4. 47° Georgii III, Session 1, cap. XXXVI An Act for the Abolition of the Slave Trade, retrieved from www.pdavis.nl/Legis_06.htm (accessed 16 Aug. 2019).

5. See for example the video 'Inside RFA Argus – the British ship on course to battle Ebola'. www.youtube.com/watch?v=IPXZh6xsu3A (accessed 7 Sept. 2018).
6. All interviewees are referred to by their first name only; all names are pseudonyms.
7. To this day 'typhoid-malaria' are named and understood as one disease by many people in Sierra Leone.
8. Ronald Ross went on to win the Nobel Prize in Medicine or Physiology for his research on *Anopheles* mosquitos and malaria transmission in 1902.

2   Colonial Mobilities and Infrastructures: The Production of (Anti)Blackness

1. When referring to the transatlantic, I do not refer only to Atlantic crossings from East to West, which have largely been centred in theorisations of Blackness, but also on crossings from North to South and South to North. These signal colonial and postcolonial mobilities, which form the basis of my analysis in this chapter.
2. Sheller (2018, p. 21) defines a mobile ontology as 'an ontology in which *movement is primary as a foundational condition of being, space, subjects, and power* [...] [an ontology that] connects multiple scales and performative sites of interaction'.
3. When speaking of 'human and material infrastructures', I use the term 'material' to denote inert objects, such as buildings or roads and consequently as distinct from human infrastructures.
4. 'The Black Man' or 'Black' is the English translation of what Mbembe in the original French version calls 'le nègre'.
5. The majority of African countries are currently excluded from visa-free travel to Europe (Passport Index, 2019).
6. The insurance policy in this case was designed to compensate the ship's owners for the unnatural deaths of enslaved Africans as they occurred during the Middle Passage (such as the throwing overboard or death as a result of a mutiny of the crew), but not for natural deaths, such as dying of thirst or starvation. M. NourbeSe Philip (Philip and Boateng, 2011) rightly questions whether dying while enslaved can ever be conceived as *natural*.
7. Colonial Development and Welfare funds were UK government grants provisioned by a series of Colonial Development Acts (1929–55). They were aimed at the economic development of Britain's colonies.
8. I was unable to find additional information on Operation Weary anywhere else.
9. At the time of its construction in 1946 the Hastings was the biggest RAF troop-carrier and freight transport aircraft of its kind (IWM, 2010).
10. Freetown International Airport was only extended with the building of a new passenger terminal in 2023. According to an article published in *Airport World* (Anonymous, 2023), this was the first new international airport terminal since the country's independence in 1961.

11. While I use Simone's terminology of 'people as infrastructure', I apply it to colonial infrastructures, rather than the fragmented, marginalised 'people as infrastructure' that Simone writes about.

12. American firm Securiport have also been tasked with ensuring security at Freetown International Airport since 2012 (Kef-Ranger, 2022).

13. There were of course many BIPOC responders to the Ebola epidemic. British-Sierra Leonean responders, in interviews, tended to reflect on the disruption of direct flights by analysing it in terms of their long-term mobility to Sierra Leone, in contrast to the more narrow, epidemic-focused analysis offered by white responders.

3   Thinking and Practising Care: Space, Risk and Racialisation in Ebola Treatment Centres

1. I lean here on Sharpe's (2016, p. 132) 'ordinary note of care' to denote an event that is extraordinary in terms of its logistical and political complexity, yet ordinary in terms of the structural, bodily and discursive violence that has characterised Black life in the wake.

2. The civil war started in the east of Sierra Leone, sweeping over from neighbouring Liberia.

3. For a more detailed discussion of family members' wish to care for their infected relatives, see Richards et al. (2019).

4. Weheliye is here quoting from D. Rodriguez, *Forced Passages* (University of Minnesota Press, 2005).

5. Hartley et al. (2017) define a CT value in Ebola testing as follows: 'the cycle threshold (CT) value was used as an inverse proxy for viral load and a cut-off of 40 was used to discriminate between positive and negative values'. As such, the lower the CT value, the higher the viral load and the higher the viral load, the higher the mortality rate.

4   Wakefulness: Epistemic Flows and Epigrammatic Antiblackness

1. The meeting was held under the Chatham House rule, whereby 'participants are free to use the information received, but neither the identity nor the affiliation of the speaker(s), nor that of any other participant, may be revealed' (Chatham House, n.d.).

2. I rely in my analysis on the video recording that has been made available online. As such, I had the opportunity to revisit the event, listen carefully to people's tone and look at their faces as they speak, something which was impossible for me to do in such detail at the time, as I was sitting at the back of the audience.

3. I draw here on my personal experience of following courses of the UCL MSc in Global Health and Development during a Cross-Disciplinary Training Scholarship I was awarded in 2018/19.

4. I agree with Chanda Prescod-Weinstein's (2020) contestation of the possibility of 'objective' researchers or 'neutral' knowledge.

5.   DFID was in existence between 1997 and 2020 when it was dissolved by Boris Johnson's Conservative government and replaced by the Foreign, Commonwealth and Development Office.

6.   This assumption has a long history, linked to antiblackness, which is touched upon among others by Grosfoguel (2013), Mignolo (2011) and other members of the Coloniality/Modernity Research Group.

References

Abdullah, I. (2017). 'God Bless WhatsApp': Neoliberal Ebola and the Struggle for Autonomous Space in Sierra Leone. In: I. Abdullah and I. Rashid, eds, *Understanding West Africa's Ebola Epidemic: Towards a Political Economy*. London: Zed Books.

Adey, P. (2010). *Aerial Life*. Chichester: John Wiley & Sons.

Ahmed, S. (2021). *Complaint!* Durham, NC: Duke University Press.

Akam, Simon, (2012). Freetown's Wood Homes a Link to Sierra Leone's Past. *Reuters*. https://uk.reuters.com/article/uk-sierraleone-architecture-idUKLNE84300 B20120504 (accessed July 2019).

Anderson, B. (2009). Affective Atmospheres. *Emotion, Space and Society* 2(2), 77–81. https://doi.org/10.1016/j.emospa.2009.08.005.

Angelou, M. (2002). *On the Pulse of Morning*. New York: Random House.

Anonymous (1901). The Liverpool Malaria Expedition. *British Medical Journal* 2(2119), 363–363.

Anonymous (2023). Freetown's New Terminal Makes History in Sierra Leone. *Airport World*, 6 March. Available at: https://airport-world.com/freetowns-new-terminal-makes-history-in-sierra-leone/ (accessed 17 Oct. 2023).

Antoine, K. (2016). 'Pushing the Edge' of Race and Gender Hegemonies through Stand-up Comedy: Performing Slavery as Anti-racist Critique. *Etnofoor* 28, 35–54.

ASHP and SCCM (American Society of Health-system Pharmacists and Society of Critical Care Medicine) (2002). Clinical Practice Guidelines for the Sustained Use of Sedatives and Analgesics in the Critically Ill Adult. *American Journal of Health-System Pharmacy* 59(2), pp. 150–178.

Bangura, J.S. (2015). Parliament Ratifies Airport Security Agreement. *Sierra Leone Concord Times*, 19 June. Available at: http://slconcordtimes.com/parliament-ratifies-airport-security-agreement/ (accessed 4 June 2018).

Barbash, F. (2014). Sierra Leone Loses Fourth Doctor to Ebola. WHO Declined to Fly Her out of the Country for Treatment. *Washington Post*, 15 Sept., Sec. Morning Mix. Available at: www.washingtonpost.com/news/morning-mix/wp/2014/09/15/sierra-leone-loses-fourth-doctor-to-ebola/ (accessed 14 June 2019).

Barrow, J., Prescod, C., Mumtaz Qureshi, I., Adi, H., Bressey, C., Carty, H. et al. (2005). *Delivering Shared Heritage: The Mayor's Commission on African and Asian Heritage*. Report. London: Greater London Authority. Available at: http://discovery.ucl.ac.uk/10002429/ (accessed June 2014).

BBC (2014). 'Ebola patients "refusing isolation" – Sierra Leone doctor', 1 Aug. www.bbc.co.uk/news/av/world-africa-28613885/ebola-patients-refusing-isolation-sierra-leone-doctor (accessed 18 May 2022).

BBC (2015). Ebola Outbreak: Sierra Leone in Lockdown. *BBC News*, 27 March. Available at: www.bbc.com/news/world-africa-32083363 (accessed 22 Jan. 2021].

Benton, A. (2014). Race and the Immuno-logics of Ebola Response in West Africa. *Somatosphere*. Available at: http://somatosphere.net/2014/race-and-the-immuno-logics-of-ebola-response-in-west-africa.html/ (accessed 27 May 2019).

Benton, A. (2015). *HIV Exceptionalism: Development through Disease in Sierra Leone*. Minneapolis, MN: University of Minnesota Press.

Benton, A. (2016a). Risky Business: Race, Nonequivalence and the Humanitarian Politics of Life. *Visual Anthropology* 29(2), 187–203. https://doi.org/10.1080/08949468.2016.1131523.

Benton, A. (2016b). African Expatriates and Race in the Anthropology of Humanitarianism. *Critical African Studies* 8(3), 266–277. https://doi.org/10.1080/21681392.2016.1244956.

Blinker, L. (2006). 'Country Environment Profile (CEP) Sierra Leone'. Cardiff, UK: Consortium Parsons Brinckerhoff. Available at: https://web.archive.org/web/20130927112254/www.sliip.org/index.php?option=com_docman&task=doc_download&gid=46 (accessed August 2019).

Booth, R. (2020). UK More Nostalgic for Empire than other Ex-colonial Powers. *The Guardian*, 11 March. Available at: www.theguardian.com/world/2020/mar/11/uk-more-nostalgic-for-empire-than-other-ex-colonial-powers.

Boyce, R. (1910). *Mosquito or Man?* London: John Murray.

Boyce, R. (1911a). *Yellow Fever and Its Prevention*. London: John Murray.

Boyce, R. (1911b). The History of Yellow Fever in West Africa. *British Medical Journal*, 1(2613), 181–185. https://doi.org/10.1136/bmj.1.2613.181.

Brand, D. (2002). *A Map to the Door of No Return: Notes to Belonging*. Toronto: Penguin Random House; Vintage Canada.

Braun, L. (2014). *Breathing Race into the Machine: The Surprising Career of the Spirometer from Plantation to Genetics*. Minneapolis, MN: University of Minnesota Press.

Bressey, C. (2006). Invisible Presence: The Whitening of the Black Community in the Historical Imagination of British Archives. *Archivaria* 61(61), 47–61.

Bressey, C. (2014). Archival Interventions: Participatory Research and Public Historical Geographies. *Journal of Historical Geography*, 46, 102–104. https://doi.org/10.1016/j.jhg.2014.07.001.

Brockett, L. (1998). The Imperial Imprint: British Colonial Towns. *New Contree* 43(6).

Calhoun, C. (2010). The Idea of Emergency: Humanitarian Action and Global (Dis)Order. In: D. Fassin and M. Pandolfi, eds, *Contemporary States of Emergency: The Politics of Military and Humanitarian Interventions*. New York: Zone Books, distributed by the MIT Press.

Casey, M. (2013). Laughter and Trauma: Making Sense of Colonial Violence. *Performing Ethos: International Journal of Ethics in Theatre & Performance* 4(1), 9–23. https://doi.org/10.1386/peet.4.1.9_1.

Chatham House (n.d.). Chatham House Rule. Chatham House – International Affairs Think Tank. Available at: www.chathamhouse.org/about-us/chatham-house-rule.

Chaulia, S. (2014). Foreign Pulse: Viral Politics. *Deccanchronicle.com*, 7 Oct. Available at: www.deccanchronicle.com/141007/commentary-columnists/article/ foreign-pulse-viral-politics (accessed 16 Apr. 2017).

Clifford, M.L. (2006). *From Slavery to Freetown: Black Loyalists after the American Revolution*. Jefferson, NC: McFarland.

Coddington, K.S. (2011). Spectral Geographies: Haunting and Everyday State Practices in Colonial and Present-day Alaska. *Social & Cultural Geography* 12(7), 743–756. https://doi.org/10.1080/14649365.2011.609411.

Cole, F. (2014). Sanitation, Disease and Public Health in Sierra Leone, West Africa, 1895–1922: Case Failure of British Colonial Health Policy. *Journal of Imperial and Commonwealth History* 43(2), 238–266. https://doi.org/10.1080/03086534. 2014.974901.

Cole, T. (2012). The White-Savior Industrial Complex. *The Atlantic*. Available at: www.theatlantic.com/international/archive/2012/03/the-white-savior-industrial-complex/254843/.

Collins, H.M. and Evans, R. (2008). *Rethinking Expertise*. Chicago: University of Chicago Press.

Cooper Owens, D. (2017). *Medical Bondage: Race, Gender, and the Origins of American Gynecology*. Athens, GA: University of Georgia Press.

Corella, M. (2018). 'I Feel Like Really Racist for Laughing': White Laughter and White Public Space in a Multiracial Classroom. In: M. Bucholtz, D.I. Casillas and J.S. Lee, eds, *Feeling It: Language, Race, and Affect in Latinx Youth Learning*. London: Routledge.

Costa Vargas, J. and Jung, M.-K. (2021). Antiblackness of the Social and the Human. In: M.-K. Jung, ed., *Antiblackness*. Durham, NC: Duke University Press. Available at: www.dukeupress.edu/antiblackness (accessed 4 May 2022).

Costa Vargas, J.H. (2018). *The Denial of Antiblackness: Multiracial Redemption and Black Suffering*. Minneapolis, MN: University of Minnesota Press.

Coultas, C. (2020). The Performativity of Monitoring and Evaluation in International Development Interventions: Building a Dialogical Case Study of Evidence-making that Situates 'the General'. *Culture & Psychology* 26(1), 96–116. https://doi.org/10.1177/1354067x19888192.

Curran, A.S. (2011). *The Anatomy of Blackness: Science and Slavery in an Age of Enlightenment*. Baltimore, MD: Johns Hopkins University Press.

Curtis, M. (2013). *Losing out: Sierra Leone's Massive Revenue Losses from Tax Incentives. Curtis Research*. Oxford: Curtis Research. Available at: http:// curtisresearch.org/publications/losing-out-sierra-leones-massive-revenue-losses-from-tax-incentives/ (accessed 1 July 2019).

Dahlgreen, W. (2014). The British Empire is 'Something to be Proud of', *YouGov*. Available at: www.yougov.co.uk/news/2014/07/26/britain-proud-its-empire (accessed 23 Oct. 2018).

Davies, S., Keogh, B., Cosford, P. and Cummings, J. (2014). 'Publications Gateway RefNo. 02266', 19 Sept. www.primarycareservices.wales.nhs.uk/sitesplus/ documents/1150/Staffing%20Letter.pdf (no longer available; accessed 31 July 2019).

Dawes, M. (n.d.). Imperial Airways – Indian Trans-Continental Airways. www. timetableimages.com. Available at: www.timetableimages.com/ttimages/iaw. htm (accessed 10 May 2022).

Deal, N.M., Mills, A.J. and Mills, J.H. (2018). Amodern and Modern Warfare in the Making of a Commercial Airline. *Management & Organizational History* 13(4), 373–396. https://doi.org/10.1080/17449359.2018.1547647.

Delph-Janiurek, T. (2001). (Un)Consensual Conversations: Betweenness, 'Material Access', Laughter and Reflexivity in Research. *Area* 33(4), 414–421. https:// doi.org/10.1111/1475-4762.00047.

Doherty, K. (2015). Journey with Maps: A Cultural Emergency Project in Freetown, Sierra Leone. *MAS Context*. Available at: www.mascontext. com/issues/25-26-legacy-spring-summer-15/journey-with-maps-a-cultural-emergency-project-in-freetown-sierra-leone/ (accessed 27 Sept. 2018).

Dorman, G. (1951). West African Wayfarings. *Flight*, 13 July, pp. 38–49.

Duffield, M. (2001). Governing the Borderlands: Decoding the Power of Aid. *Disasters* 25(4), 308–320. https://doi.org/10.1111/1467-7717.00180.

Duffield, M. (2008). Global Civil War: The Non-insured, International Containment and Post-interventionary Society. *Journal of Refugee Studies* 21(2). https:// doi.org/10.1093/jrs/femo4.

Dym, H. and Ogle, O. (2011). *Oral Surgery for the General Dentist, An Issue of Dental Clinics*. Amsterdam: Elsevier Health Sciences.

Evans, D.K., Goldstein, M. and Popova, A. (2015). Health-care Worker Mortality and the Legacy of the Ebola Epidemic. *Lancet Global Health* 3(8), e439–e440. https://doi.org/10.1016/S2214-109X(15)00065-0.

Fanon, F. (1965). *A Dying Colonialism*. New York: Grove Press.

Fanon, F. (1988 [1952]). *Toward the African Revolution: Political Essays*. New York: Grove Press.

Fanon, F. (2011). *Oeuvres*. Paris: Découverte.

Farmer, A. (2018). Archiving While Black. *Chronicle of Higher Education*. Available at: www.chronicle.com/article/Archiving-While-Black/243981 (accessed 13 June 2019).

Farmer, P. (2014). Diary. *London Review of Books*, 23 Oct.

Fassin, D. (2007). Humanitarianism as a Politics of Life. *Public Culture* 19(3), 499–520. https://doi.org/10.1215/08992363-2007-007.

Ferme, M.C. (2001). *The Underneath of Things*. Berkeley, CA: University of California Press.

Ferreira da Silva, D. (2015). Before Man: Sylvia Wynter's Rewriting of the Modern Episteme. In: K. McKittrick, ed., *Sylvia Wynter: On Being Human as Praxis*. Durham, NC: Duke University Press.

Frankfurter, R., Kardas-Nelson, M., Benton, A., Barrie, M.B., Dibba, Y., Farmer, P. et al. (2019). Indirect Rule Redux: The Political Economy of Diamond Mining and its Relation to the Ebola Outbreak in Kono District, Sierra Leone. *Review of African Political Economy* 45(158), 522–540. https://doi.org/10.1080/0305624 4.2018.1547188.

Frenkel, S. and Western, J. (1988). Pretext or Prophylaxis? Racial Segregation and Malarial Mosquitos in a British Tropical Colony: Sierra Leone.

Annals of the Association of American Geographers 78(2), 211–228. https://doi.org/10.1111/j.1467-8306.1988.tb00203.x.

Fuentes, M.J. (2018). *Disposessed Lives: Enslaved Women, Violence, and the Archive.* Reprint edn. Philadelphia, PA: University of Pennsylvania Press.

Fyfe, C. (1961). Four Sierra Leone Recaptives. *Journal of African History* 2(1), 77–85. https://doi.org/10.1017/s0021853700002152.

Fyfe, C. (1962). *A History of Sierra Leone.* London: Oxford University Press.

Gberie, L. (2017). Opinion: Sierra Leone's Disaster Was Caused by Neglect, Not Nature. *The New York Times*, 20 Aug. Available at: www.nytimes.com/2017/08/20/opinion/sierra-leones-sugarloaf-mudslide.html (accessed May 2019).

Gilmore, R.W. (2002). Fatal Couplings of Power and Difference: Notes on Racism and Geography. *Professional Geographer* 54(1), 15–24. https://doi.org/10.1111/0033-0124.00310.

Global Fund (2017). *Rebuilding Health Care in the Shadow of Ebola – Sierra Leone.* reliefweb.int. Available at: https://reliefweb.int/report/sierra-leone/rebuilding-health-care-shadow-ebola (accessed 13 May 2019).

Grosfoguel, R. (2013). The Structure of Knowledge in Westernized Universities: Epistemic Racism/Sexism and the Four Genocides/Epistemicides of the Long 16th Century. *Human Architecture: Journal of the Sociology of Self-Knowledge* 11(1). Available at: https://scholarworks.umb.edu/humanarchitecture/vol11/iss1/8 (accessed 2 Aug. 2023).

Hall, C., Draper, N., McClelland, K., Donington, K. and Lang, R. (2014). *Legacies of British Slave-ownership Colonial Slavery and the Formation of Victorian Britain.* Cambridge: Cambridge University Press.

Harker, J. (2014). Why are Western Health Workers with Ebola Flown Out, but Locals Left to Die? *The Guardian.* 15 Sept. Available at: www.theguardian.com/commentisfree/2014/sep/15/ebola-doctor-death-olivet-buck-sierra-leone (accessed 14 Dec. 2022).

Hartley, M.-A., Young, A., Tran, A.-M., Okoni-Williams, H.H., Suma, M., Mancuso, B. et al. (2017). Predicting Ebola Severity: A Clinical Prioritization Score for Ebola Virus Disease. *PLOS Neglected Tropical Diseases* 11(2), e0005265. https://doi.org/10.1371/journal.pntd.0005265.

Hartman, S.V. (1997). *Scenes of Subjection: Terror, Slavery, and Self-making in Nineteenth-century America.* New York: Oxford University Press.

Hartman, S.V. (2020). *Wayward Lives, Beautiful Experiments: Intimate Histories of Social Upheaval.* New York: W.W. Norton.

Hodge J.M. (2007). *Triumph of the Expert: Agrarian Doctrines of Development and the Legacies of British Colonialism.* Athens, OH: Ohio University Press.

Ingham, E.G. and Clarkson, T. (1894). *Sierra Leone after a Hundred Years.* London: Seeley.

IWM (Imperial War Museums) (2010). Handley Page Hastings C1A. Available at: http://www.iwm.org.uk/collections/item/object/70000172 (accessed 26 August 2019).

Jacobi, J., Fraser, G.L., Coursin, D.B., Riker, R.R., Fontaine, D., Wittbrodt, E.T. et al. (2002). Clinical Practice Guidelines for the Sustained Use of Sedatives and Analgesics in the Critically Ill Adult. *Critical Care Medicine* 30(1), 119–141. https://doi.org/10.1097/00003246-200201000-00020.

Johnson, R. (2010). 'An All-white Institution': Defending Private Practice and the Formation of the West African Medical Staff. *Medical History* 54(2), 237–254. https://doi.org/10.1017/s0025727300006736.

Jolie, A. (2021). Malone Mukwende Has a Plan to Close the Racial Gap in Medical Care. *Time*. Available at: https://time.com/6074742/angelina-jolie-malone-mukwende-hutano-mind-the-gap/ (accessed 26 Feb. 2023).

Jpatokal (2009). English: Map of Scheduled Airline Traffic around the World, circa June 2009. Contains 54317 routes, rendered at 25% transparency. Wikimedia Commons. Available at: https://commons.wikimedia.org/wiki/File:World-airline-routemap-2009.png (accessed May 2022).

Kamara, S. (2018). Sierra Leone Is Deeply Grateful for the Aid, Britain – But Now Let's Trade. BrexitCentral. Available at: https://brexitcentral.com/sierra-leone-deeply-grateful-aid-britain-now-lets-trade/ (accessed 26 Oct. 2023).

Kandeh, J.D. (1992). Politicization of Ethnic Identities in Sierra Leone. *African Studies Review* 35(1), 81. https://doi.org/10.2307/524446.

Kef-Ranger, A. (2022). Securiport's $25 Security Fee Levied on Travelers is Justifiable & Tenable. *The Calabash Newspaper*, 1 July. Available at: https://thecalabashnewspaper.com/securiports-25-security-fee-levied-on-travelers-is-justifiable-tenable/ (accessed 26 Oct. 2023).

King, T.L. (2019). *The Black Shoals: Offshore Formations of Black and Native Studies*. Durham, NC: Duke University Press.

Koutroumpi, S. (2020). *Understanding Thermal Conditions, Thermal Comfort and Adaptive Behaviours in Naturally Ventilated Multi-patient Wards in Connaught Hospital, Freetown, Sierra Leone*. Thesis. Available at: www.mybib.com/#/projects/eeXrMJ/citations/new/thesis (accessed 10 May 2022).

KSLP (2019). *Connaught Hospital – King's Sierra Leone Partnership*. Available at: https://kslp.org.uk/partners/connaught-hospital/ (accessed May 2019).

Latour, B. (1993). *The Pasteurization of France*. Cambridge, MA: Harvard University Press.

Legg, S. (2007). *Spaces of Colonialism*. Malden, MA: Blackwell Publishing.

Leigh, J. (2016). *A History of St. Edward's Church*. Createspace Independent Publishing Platform.

Lewis, R. (1954). *Sierra Leone: A Modern Portrait*. London: Her Majesty's Stationery Office (Corona Library).

Lipton, J. (2017). 'Black' and 'White' Death: Burials in a Time of Ebola in Freetown, Sierra Leone. *Journal of the Royal Anthropological Institute* 23(4), 801–819. https://doi.org/10.1111/1467-9655.12696.

Logistics Cluster (2022). *2.2.2 Sierra Leone Kenema National Airfield | Digital Logistics Capacity Assessments*. dlca.logcluster.org. Available at: https://dlca.logcluster.org/222-sierra-leone-kenema-national-airfield (accessed 17 Oct. 2023).

LSHTM (London School of Hygiene and Tropical Medicine) (2017). Global Response to Ebola meeting – 25 Nov 2015. Vimeo. Available at: https://vimeo.com/204212744. (accessed 26 Oct. 2023).

Martinez, J.S. (2012). The Courts of Mixed Commission for the Abolition of the Slave Trade. In: *The Slave Trade and the Origins of International Human Rights*

Law. Oxford: Oxford University Press, pp. 67–98. https://doi.org/10.1093/acprof:osobl/9780195391626.003.0004.

Maslen, R. (2012). British Airways Resumes Monrovia Link | *Aviation Week Network*. aviationweek.com. Available at: www.routesonline.com/news/29/breaking-news/162494/british-airways-resumes-monrovia-link/ (accessed 26 Oct. 2023).

Massaquoi, M. (2016). British Airways Reinstate Please Direct Flights to Sierra Leone and Liberia. Change.org. Available at: www.change.org/p/british-airways-p-o-box365-harmonds-worth-middlesex-ub7-ogb-british-airways-reinstate-please-direct-flights-to-sierra-leone-and-liberia (accessed 26 Oct. 2023).

Massaquoi, M. (2018). Petition Update. Change.org. Available at: www.change.org/p/british-airways-p-o-box365-harmonds-worth-middlesex-ub7-ogb-british-airways-reinstate-please-direct-flights-to-sierra-leone-and-liberia/u/22894202 (accessed 26 Oct. 2023).

Massumi, B. (2015). *The Politics of Affect*. Cambridge: Polity.

Mbembe, A. (2001). *On the Postcolony*. Berkeley, CA: University of California Press.

Mbembe, J.-A. (2017). *Critique of Black Reason*, trans. L. Dubois. Durham, NC: Duke University Press.

McKittrick, K. (2006). *Demonic Grounds: Black Women and the Cartographies of Struggle*. Minneapolis, MN: University of Minnesota Press.

McKittrick, K. (2021). *Dear Science and Other Stories*. Durham, NC: Duke University Press.

Mignolo, W.D. (2009). Epistemic Disobedience, Independent Thought and Decolonial Freedom. *Theory, Culture & Society* 26(7–8), 159–181. https://doi.org/10.1177/0263276409349275.

Mignolo, W. (2011). *The Darker Side of Western Modernity: Global Futures, Decolonial Options*. Durham, NC: Duke University Press.

Mignolo, W.D. (2015). Sylvia Wynter: What Does It Mean to Be Human? In: K. McKittrick, ed., *Sylvia Wynter: On Being Human as Praxis*. Durham, NC: Duke University Press.

Mol, A. (2002). *The Body Multiple: Ontology in Medical Practice*. Durham: Duke University Press.

Morrison, T. (1987). *Beloved*. London: Chatto & Windus.

Mukwende, M., Tamony, P. and Turner, M. (2020). *Mind the Gap: A Handbook of Clinical Signs in Black and Brown Skin*. London: St George's University. Available at: www.blackandbrownskin.co.uk/mindthegap (accessed 4 May 2022).

Nading, A.M. (2017). Local Biologies, Leaky Things, and the Chemical Infrastructure of Global Health. *Medical Anthropology* 36(2), 141–156. https://doi.org/10.1080/01459740.2016.1186672.

NHGRI (2018). Genetics vs. Genomics Fact Sheet, National Human Genome Research Institute. Available at: https://www.genome.gov/about-genomics/factsheets/Genetics-vs-Genomics (accessed 16 May 2022).

Noxolo, P. (2006). Claims: A Postcolonial Geographical Critique of 'Partnership' in Britain's Development Discourse. *Singapore Journal of Tropical Geography* 27(3), 254–269. https://doi.org/10.1111/j.1467-9493.2006.00261.x.

Nuttall, S. (2009). *Entanglement*. Johannesburg: Wits University Press.

Nye, E. and Gibson, M. (1997). *Ronald Ross: Malariologist and Polymath: A Biography*. London: Springer.

O'Dempsey, T. (2017). Failing Dr Khan. In: M. Hofman and S. Au, eds, *The Politics of Fear*. Oxford: Oxford University Press.

O'Hare, B. (2015). Weak Health Systems and Ebola. *Lancet Global Health* 3(2), e71–e72. https://doi.org/10.1016/s2214-109x(14)70369-9.

Olufemi, L. (2021). *Experiments in Imagining Otherwise*. Maidstone: Hajar Press.

Olusoga, D. (2016). *Black and British: A Forgotten History*. London: Pan Macmillan.

PAC (Public Accounts Committee) (2015). *The UK's Response to the Outbreak of Ebola Virus Disease in West Africa – Public Accounts Committee*. London: House of Commons. Available at: https://publications.parliament.uk/pa/cm201415/cmselect/cmpubacc/868/86806.htm#note4 (accessed 1 July 2019).

Passport Index (2019). Global Passport Power Rank | Passport Index 2019, Passport Index – All the world's passports in one place. Available at: https://www.passportindex.org/byRank.php (accessed 26 August 2019).

Patterson, O. (1982). *Slavery and Social Death: A Comparative Study*. Cambridge, MA: Harvard University Press.

Pauwels, M. (2021). White Laughter, Black Pain? On the Comic and Parodic Enactment of Racial-colonial Stereotypes. In: E. Vanderheiden and C.-H. Mayer, eds, *The Palgrave Handbook of Humour Research*. Cham, Switzerland: Springer International Publishing, pp. 227–241. https://doi.org/10.1007/978-3-030-78280-1_12.

Philip, M.N. and Boateng, S.A. (2011). *Zong!* Middletown, CT: Wesleyan University Press.

Pickens, T.A. (2019). *Black Madness :: Mad Blackness*. Durham, NC: Duke University Press.

Piepzna-Samarasinha, L.L. (2018). *Care Work: Dreaming Disability Justice*. Vancouver: Arsenal Pulp Press.

Pierre, J. (2013). *The Predicament of Blackness: Postcolonial Ghana and the Politics of Race*. Chicago: University of Chicago Press.

Piot, P. (2012). *No Time to Lose: A Life in Pursuit of Deadly Viruses*. 1st edn. New York: W.W. Norton.

Pollack, A. (2014). Opting against Ebola Drug for Ill African Doctor. *The New York Times*, 12 Aug. Available at: www.nytimes.com/2014/08/13/world/africa/ebola.html (accessed 14 Jun. 2016).

Prescod-Weinstein, C. (2020). Making Black Women Scientists under White Empiricism: The Racialization of Epistemology in Physics. *Signs: Journal of Women in Culture and Society* 45(2), 421–447. https://doi.org/10.1086/704991.

Prince of Wales, Salmond, G., Churchill, W., Amery, C., Haig, E. and Trenchard, H. (1920). Imperial Air Routes: Discussion. *The Geographical Journal* 55(4), 263–70.

Purvis, K. (2014). Ebola: The Story of the Sierra Leone Diaspora Response that No One is Telling. *The Guardian*. Available at: www.theguardian.com/global-development-professionals-network/2014/oct/09/ebola-response-diaspora-sierra-leone (accessed 23 May 2021).

Raghuram, P., Madge, C. and Noxolo, P. (2009). Rethinking Responsibility and Care for a Postcolonial World. *Geoforum* 40(1), 5–13. https://doi.org/10.1016/j.geoforum.2008.07.007.

Rankin, F.H. (1836). *The White Man's Grave: A Visit to Sierra Leone, in 1834*. London: R. Bentley.

RedR (2010). About RedR: Humanitarian Training for NGOs and Relief Workers Worldwide. RedR. Available at: www.redr.org.uk/About.

RedR (n.d.). Training Medical Staff Deployed to Fight Ebola in West Africa. RedR. Available at: www.redr.org.uk/Our-Work/Previous-Projects/Ebola-(2015-2016) (accessed 26 Oct. 2023).

Reuters Staff (2014). Netherlands to Evacuate Two Doctors who Had Contact with Ebola Victims. *Reuters*, 12 Sept. Available at: www.reuters.com/article/uk-health-ebola-dutch-idUKKBN0H70UZ20140912 (accessed 26 Oct. 2023).

Richards, P. (2016). *Ebola: How a People's Science Helped End an Epidemic*. London: Zed Books.

Richards, P., Mokuwa, E., Welmers, P., Maat, H. and Beisel, U. (2019). Trust, and Distrust, of Ebola Treatment Centers: A Case-study from Sierra Leone. *PLOS ONE* 14(12), e0224511. https://doi.org/10.1371/journal.pone.0224511.

Richardson, E.T., McGinnis, T. and Frankfurter, R. (2019). Ebola and the Narrative of Mistrust. *BMJ Global Health* 4(6), e001932. https://doi.org/10.1136/bmjgh-2019-001932.

Robinson, H. (2017). Black Women's Voices and the Archive. *Black Perspectives*. Available at: www.aaihs.org/black-womens-voices-and-the-archive/ (accessed 13 June 2019).

Rodney, W. (1980). *A History of the Upper Guinea Coast, 1545–1800*. New York: Monthly Review Press.

Rogers, T. (2015). British Airways return to Sierra Leone. *38degrees.org.uk*. Available at: https://you.38degrees.org.uk/petitions/british-airways-return-to-sierra-leone (accessed 26 Oct. 2023).

Royal Geographical Society (Great Britain) (RGS) (1836). List of Members. *Journal of the Royal Geographical Society* 7, xxviii.

Royal Society (2019). About us | History of the Royal Society | Royal Society. royalsociety.org. Available at: https://royalsociety.org/about-us/.

Rubyan-Ling, D. (2019). Diaspora Mobilization and the Politics of Loyalty in the Time of Ebola: Evidence from the Sierra Leonean Diaspora in the UK. *Global Networks* 19(2), 218–237. https://doi.org/10.1111/glob.12213.

Saini, A. (2019). *Superior: The Return of Race science*. London: Fourth Estate.

Sankoh, F.P., Yan, X. and Tran, Q. (2013). Environmental and Health Impact of Solid Waste Disposal in Developing Cities: A Case Study of Granville Brook Dumpsite, Freetown, Sierra Leone. *Journal of Environmental Protection* 4(7), 665–670. https://doi.org/10.4236/jep.2013.47076.

Seeley, S. (2016). Beyond the American Colonization Society. *History Compass* 14(3), 93–104. https://doi.org/10.1111/hic3.12302.

Sharpe, C. (2016). *In the Wake: On Blackness and Being*. Durham, NC: Duke University Press.

Sharpe, C. (2018). 'And to Survive'. *Small Axe: A Caribbean Journal of Criticism* 22(3), 171–180. https://doi.org/10.1215/07990537-7249304.

Shaw, R. (2002). *Memories of the Slave Trade: Ritual and the Historical Imagination in Sierra Leone*. Chicago: University of Chicago Press.

Sheller, M. (2018). *Mobility Justice: The Politics of Movement in an Age of Extremes.* London: Verso.

Sheppard, E. (2002). The Spaces and Times of Globalization: Place, Scale, Networks, and Positionality. *Economic Geography* 78(3), 307. https://doi. org/10.2307/4140812.

Sibthorpe, A.B.C. (1970). The history of Sierra Leone. 4th edn. London: Frank Cass and Co.

Sierra Leone Company (1791). *Substance of the Report from the Court of Directors to the General Court of the Sierra Leone Company.* London: Sierra Leone Company. Available at: www.sierra-leone.org/Books/Substance_of_the_report_of_the_court_of-1791.pdf (accessed 5 July 2019).

Simone, A. (2004). People as Infrastructure: Intersecting Fragments in Johannesburg. *Public Culture* 16(3), 407–429. https://doi.org/10.1215/08992363-16-3-407.

Sowemimo, A. (2023). *Divided.* London: Profile Books.

Smilie, I., Gberie, L. and Hazleton, R. (2000). *The Heart of the Matter: Sierra Leone, Diamonds and Human Security.* Ottawa: Partnership Africa Canada.

Spencer, S. (2015). 'Invisible Enemy' – Translating Ebola Prevention and Control Measures in Sierra Leone. In: U. Engel and R. Rottenburg, eds, *Working Papers of the Priority Programme 1448 of the German Research Foundation.* Leipzig and Halle: German Research Foundation, pp. 1–19.

Spitzer, L. (1968). The Mosquito and Segregation in Sierra Leone. *Canadian Journal of African Studies* 2(1), 49–61. https://doi.org/10.1080/00083968.1968.108 03498.

Stoler, A.L. (2013). *Imperial Debris: On Ruins and Ruination.* Durham, NC: Duke University Press.

Stoler, A.L. (2016). *Duress: Imperial Durabilities in Our Times.* Durham, NC: Duke University Press.

Stone, M.-L. (2012). Freetown Cabins Recall Birth of Colony – in Pictures. *The Guardian*, 3 May. Available at: www.theguardian.com/world/gallery/2012/may/03/freetown-sierra-leone-architecture-pictures (accessed 26 Oct. 2023).

Street, A. (2011). Affective Infrastructure. *Space and Culture* 15(1), 44–56. https://doi.org/10.1177/1206331211426061.

Street, A. (2014). *Biomedicine in an Unstable Place: Infrastructure and Personhood in a Papua New Guinean Hospital.* Durham, NC: Duke University Press.

Suzuki, Y. (2018). The Good Farmer: Morality, Expertise, and Articulations of Whiteness in Zimbabwe. *Anthropological Forum* 28(1), 74–88. https://doi.org/10. 1080/00664677.2018.1429252.

Tarawallie, I. (n.d.). Gambia Bird Begins London to Freetown Air Service. Sierra Leone News, This is Sierra Leone, All about Sierra Leone and Sierra Leone News. Available at: www.thisissierraleone.com/gambia-bird-begins-london-to-freetown-air-service (accessed 2 Jun. 2018).

Taylor, L. (1902). Sanitary Work in West Africa. *British Medical Journal* 2(2177), 852–54.

The New Humanitarian (2014). A Tribute to Two Ebola Heroes. Available at: www.thenewhumanitarian.org/feature/2014/08/19/tribute-two-ebola-heroes (accessed 6 Sept. 2021).

Thomas, A.R. (2019a). Ebola in Sierra Leone and the Death of Dr. Sheikh Umarr Khan – Five Years on, No Answers. *The Sierra Leone Telegraph*. Available at: www.thesierraleonetelegraph.com/ebola-in-sierra-leone-and-the-death-of-dr-sheikh-umarr-khan-five-years-on-no-answers/ (accessed 30 July 2019).

Thomas, A.R. (2019b). Is Sierra Leone Likely to See the Return of Direct London to Freetown Flights Anytime Soon? *The Sierra Leone Telegraph*. Available at: www.thesierraleonetelegraph.com/is-sierra-leone-likely-to-see-the-return-of-direct-london-to-freetown-flights-anytime-soon/ (accessed 27 Aug. 2021).

Tinsley, R. (2018). *The Lingering Legacy of Ebola in Sierra Leone*. Open Democracy. Available at: www.opendemocracy.net/en/lingering-legacy-of-ebola-in-sierra-leone/ (accessed 26 Oct. 2023).

Trans-Atlantic Slave Trade Database (2013). *Trans-Atlantic Slave Trade – Database*. www.slavevoyages.org. Available at: http://slavevoyages.org/voyage/search (accessed 26 Oct. 2023).

Tuck, E. and Yang, K.W. (2012). Decolonization is Not a Metaphor. *Decolonization: Indigeneity, Education & Society* 1(1), 1–40.

van Roekel, E. (2016). Uncomfortable Laughter. Reflections on Violence, Humour and Immorality in Argentina. *Etnofoor* 28(1), 55–74.

Vinck, P., Pham, P.N., Bindu, K.K., Bedford, J. and Nilles, E.J. (2019). Institutional Trust and Misinformation in the Response to the 2018–19 Ebola Outbreak in North Kivu, DR Congo: A Population-based Survey. *Lancet Infectious Diseases* 19(5), 529–536. https://doi.org/10.1016/s1473-3099(19)30063-5.

Weheliye, A.G. (2015). *Habeas Viscus Racializing Assemblages, Biopolitics, and Black Feminist Theories of the Human*. Durham, NC: Duke University Press.

White, L. (2000). *Speaking with Vampires*. Berkeley, CA: University of California Press.

WHO (2015). *Ebola in Sierra Leone: A Slow Start to an Outbreak that Eventually Outpaced All Others*. World Health Organization. https://doi.org/entity/csr/disease/ebola/one-year-report/sierra-leone/en/index.html.

Wilson, E.G. (1976). *The Loyal Blacks*. New York: Capricorn Books.

Wynter, S. (1994). No Humans Involved: An Open Letter to My Colleagues. *Forum N.H.I. Knowledge for the Twenty-first Century* 1(1), 42–73.

Wynter, S. (2001). Towards the Sociogenic Principle: Fanon, Identity, the Puzzle of Conscious Experience, and What It Is Like to Be 'Black'. In: A. Gomez-Moriana and M. Duran-Cogan, eds, *National Identities and Socio-political Changes in Latin America*. London: Routledge.

Wynter, S. (2003). Unsettling the Coloniality of Being/Power/Truth/Freedom: Towards the Human, After Man, Its Overrepresentation – An Argument. *CR: The New Centennial Review* 3(3), 257–337. https://doi.org/10.1353/ncr.2004.0015.

Wynter, S. (2006). 'PROUD FLESH Inter/Views: Sylvia Wynter', *ProudFlesh: New Afrikan Journal of Culture, Politics and Consciousness*, issue 4, pp. 1–36.

Yusoff, K. (2018). *A Billion Black Anthropocenes or None*. Minneapolis, MN: University of Minnesota Press.

Zook, M.A. and Brunn, S.D. (2006). From Podes to Antipodes: Positionalities and Global Airline Geographies. *Annals of the Association of American Geographers* 96(3), 471–490. https://doi.org/10.1111/j.1467-8306.2006.00701.x.

Archival Sources

The National Archives (TNA) in Kew

Archival reference	Item description
CO937/510	Applications and descriptions of the development of Lungi and Kenema airports
CO1045/515	Sierra Leone correspondence and papers
CO937/262	Development of Lingi Airport at Freetown, Sierra Leone, 1953
CO937/544	Sierra Leone. Colonial Office and Commonwealth Office: Communication Department: Original Correspondence. Civil Aviation. 1960
CO271/17	Government Gazettes, 1919
CO1071/323	Sierra Leone colonial reports, 1906–24
CO270/45	Administration Reports, 1910–13
WO1/352	Africa and the Atlantic Islands. iv. Sierra Leone. Sierra Leone Company, 1800–1807
CO1069/88/20	Sierra Leone. Photograph No. 19: 'The Colonial Hospital, southern view', 1871
CO1069/88/22	Sierra Leone. Photograph No. 21: 'The Colonial Hospital, eastern view', 1871
CO1069/88/181	Sierra Leone. Photograph No. 48: Colonial Secretary's Bungalow
CO1069/88/241	Sierra Leone. 'Visit of their Royal Highness's the Duke and Duchess of Connaught to Sierra Leone', 15th December 1910.

The Wellcome Trust Archives

Reference	Description
GC/59/A	Yellow Fever (West Africa) Commission 1913
.b21355113	Yellow Fever and its Prevention: A Manual for Medical Students and Practitioners by Rubert W. Boyce
LA/BOY	Mosquito or Man? The Conquest of the Tropical World by Rubert W. Boyce
EPB RAMC	The White Man's Grave: A Visit to Sierra Leone, in 1834 by F. Harrison Rankin (1836)

British Medical Journal Archives

Anonymous. (1901). The Liverpool Malaria Expedition. *British Medical Journal* 2(2119), 363–363.

Boyce, R. (1911b). The History of Yellow Fever in West Africa. *British Medical Journal* 1(2613), 181–185.

Taylor, L. (1902). Sanitary Work in West Africa. *British Medical Journal* 2(2177), 852–854.

Royal Geographical Society Archives

Royal Geographical Society (Great Britain) (1836). *Journal of the Royal Geographical Society* 7.

Prince of Wales, Salmond, G., Churchill, W., Colonel Amery, Haig, E. and Trenchard, H. (1920). Imperial Air Routes: Discussion. *The Geographical Journal* 55(4), 263–270.

Index

ill refers to an illustration; *n* to a note

38degrees.com (petition) 81

Accra 47
Act for the Abolition of the Slave
    Trade (1833) 38
Act for the Abolition of the Slave
    Trade (1807) 32, 33, 38, 96
Adey, Peter 67, 140–1
aeromobility 62, 67, 71, 73–84, 140–1
    infrastructure in 73–6
    segregation in 69–70
Africa
    colonisation of 20, 24, 30, 133
    and transport mobilities 62–70
    see also sub-Saharan Africa; West
        Africa and specific countries
African diaspora 14
African Minerals Company 129
Africanness 11–12, 154
afro-pessimism 8
Ahmed, Sara 136
AIDS *see* HIV/AIDS
American Colonization Society (ACS)
    133
American embassy, Hill Station 31
American War of Independence 25–6
Angelou, Maya *On the Pulse of
    Morning* 16–17
Annual Medical Report on Sierra
    Leone (1913) 38
Anthropocene 14
antiblackness xvii–xviii, 10–11, 16,
    23, 32, 125, 139–40
    epigrammatic realities of 125, 126,
        140
    and weather 11, 23, 41–2, 45, 51
archives 95, 135–40
    racist attitudes of staff 136–40

atherosclerosis 94, 104, 118
atmosphere 42, 52
atopic dermatitis xviii

Baldry, Sir Tony 78
Banana Islands 22
Benton, Adia 7, 125, 141, 146, 150
biomedical care 37, 39–41, 52–4, 56,
    95, 98–9, 100–2, 114, 121–2, 153
biomedicine 10–12, 33, 35, 52–5,
    99–102
BIPOC (disabled, queer, women,
    Black, Indigenous, Peoples of
    Colour) 10, 96, 114, 136
Black African people
    agency of 3, 4–5, 6, 8, 27, 73, 135
    mortality rate of 14, 40
Black colonial settlers 133
Black feminism 103
Black mobile ontologies 58–60, 62,
    64, 69–70, 84, 89
Black Studies xix, 5, 8, 9–10, 15–16,
    89, 95, 134, 158
Black women 135
Blackness 59, 64–5, 69–70, 79, 147
    see also antiblackness
Boyce, Rupert 43, 44–6, 66, 141
    Yellow Fever and Its Prevention 43
Brand, Dionne *A Map to the Door of
    No Return* 16
Braun, Lundy 12
Bressey, Caroline 125, 135, 155
British Airways, suspension of flights
    to Sierra Leone 61, 71, 80, 81–9
British colonialism 20, 25–6, 133–4,
    125
    British attitudes to 132–3, 142
British Medical Journal 44, 46, 47

British Midlands International (bmi) 80
British Overseas Airways Corporation (BOAC) 67, 69, 77–8, 80
Brussels Airways 80, 82–3, 87, 88
Buck, Dr Olivet 3–4, 71, 144
Bunce Island landing dock 64*ill*

care practice 92–158
    segregation in 39–41
    sharing in 111–8, 120–2
    violence in 32, 94–8, 99–100, 114, 122
    see also biomedical care; health care
Casas, Bartolomé de las 9
Centers for Disease Control (CDCs) 2
Césaire, Aimé 9
change.org (petition) 81–2
Chatham House 127, 162*n*1
Chaulia, Sreeram 129
child slaves 35
chlorine 54–5, 110–1, 119–20
Christianity 100–1
Churchill, Winston 67
Clarkson, John 26
Coddington, K.S. 53
Cole, Teju 5
Colonial Hospital 28*ill*, 37–8, 39–40
colonial infrastructures 62, 79, 90, 156
colonial mobilities 61–71, 74–80, 88
colonialism 133–4, 140, 149
    epigrammatic attitudes to 126, 134, 141, 147, 155, 158
    ruination by 5, 27, 28
    see also British colonialism; neo-colonialism; Portuguese colonialism
Concern Worldwide (NGO) xv
Connaught, Arthur, Duke of Connaught 32, 38
Connaught Hospital 32–3, 36, 37*ill*, 38–9, 55, 116–7, 120
Corella, Meghan 129
Costa Vargas, João and M.K. Jung 9, 11, 14

cotton plantations, and slavery xvii
Courts of Mixed Commission 33, 34, 63
Covid-19 pandemic 14, 156
craniology 12
Cruz, Alex 80
Curran, Andrew 10

Daily Mail 88
Davies, Dame Sally 40–1
De Beers company 75
Decolonising Global Health movement 16, 160*n*3
Delph-Janiurek, T. 128–9
Democratic Republic of the Congo 52, 99, 143
Department for International Development (DFID) 142, 163*n*5
diamond mining 74–5
diazepam 117–8
disabled people 10, 93, 96, 99
Dorman, Geoffrey 68–9

Ebola cemetery xv
Ebola epidemic xvii, 1–5
    patients' lack of trust in medical services 53–6
    and risk 114–21
    rumour and conspiracy theories about 53–6, 97–8
    status of 106–8
Ebola Holding Units (EHUs) 102, 104, 109, 112–3, 115–7, 120
Ebola Treatment Centres (ETCs) 48–50, 98, 103, 105–6
    brick buildings 50
    map 105*ill*
    orange zones 105
    red zones 49–51, 105–6, 113
    risks in 105–6, 109–13
    segregation in 48, 103–4, 112
epistemic disobedience 15, 16
epistemic spaces 126, 130
European knowledge 15, 16, 102, 124, 146
European medicine 12–13
    see also biomedicine

EVD *see* Ebola

Fanon, Frantz 9, 30, 34, 133
Fernando Po Island 44
Flight (magazine) 68
flow 60, 66, 111–3
  epistemic 124, 140, 147, 155
  regulation of 109–13
France, response to Ebola 132
Freetown 8–9, 24–32, 66
  air transport links to colonies 68
  colonial place names in 24–5
  colonial urban design of 27–32,
    29*ill*, 41
  and disease 31, 45
  map (1913) 28*ill*
  social and racial segregation in 27,
    30, 39
  transport links with London 66, 80
Freetown International Airport 78–9,
    161*n*10
Frenkel, S. and J. Western 97
Fuentes, Marisa J. 125, 135, 155
Fyfe, Christopher 30, 33

Gamba Bird Airline 80, 82, 84, 87
Garner, Margaret 22
Gaza 156
germ theory 45
Germany, racism in xiii–xv
Ghana 68
Ghana Airways 77
Gilmore, Ruth Wilson 103
global health 4–5, 7, 13–15, 121, 127,
    131, 157–8
Granville Brooke 24–5
Gregson v. Gilbert 72–3
Guinea 53, 60, 128, 132, 140
gynaecology 12

Hammond, Philip 132
Hartman, Saidiya 9
  *Wayward Lives, Beautiful Experi-
    ments* 95
Harvard University 126
hauntings 53, 56–7
Havelock, Sir Arthur 46

health care 92–102, 116–7, 121–2
  segregation in 39–41, 46–8
  violence in 94, 97–9, 114
health care workers 41, 103, 143
  deaths from Ebola 103–4
  evacuation of 3, 71, 115
  racist treatment of 48–9, 142
  repatriation of 143
  risks to 105–6, 109–13
  volunteers 142–5
Hill Station, Freetown 28–32, 29*ill*, 39
  health conditions in 30–1
  ruination of 32
HIV/AIDS xiv–xv, 142
Hodge, Joseph Morgan 125
human beings 10, 13, 100–1
human infrastructures 74, 76, 78
humanitarian imperialism 26, 97
humanitarian intervention 101–2,
    141–2

Imperial Airways 67
  flight route map (1931) 68*ill*
independence movements 76–7
infection protection and control
    (IPC) 111, 122
infrastructures 60–3, 73–143
  see also aeromobility; colonial
    infrastructures; human infra-
    structures; transport
infrastructures
Ingham, Ernest Graham 26
International Military Advisory and
    Training Team (IMATT) 31
International SOS company 2

Johannesburg 76
Johnson, Dr Oliver 53–4

Kailahun 1, 98
Kenema airfield 74–5, 78
Kenema Government Hospital 1
Kent, Freetown 21*ill*, 22
Kenya 52
Keogh, Sir Bruce 41
Kerry Town ETC 19, 40–1, 148
  ruination of 19

Khan, Dr 1-2, 4, 71
King, Tiffany Lethabo 15
King-Harman, Charles 30
King's Yard 33, 34, 35-6, 37*ill*, 63-4
Kingsley, Mary 59
Koroma, Ernest Bai 3

Lancet, The 127, 129
laughter 128-30, 139-40
  white laughter 129-30
Lewis, Roy *Sierra Leone: a Modern
  Portrait* 30
Liberated African Hospital 37
Liberia 2, 132, 133, 140
Lion Heart Medical Centre 3
Lipton, Jonah 52-3
Liverpool School of Tropical
  Medicine 43, 46
London Mining Company 129
London School of Hygiene and
  Tropical Medicine 126
Lumley Government Hospital 3
Lungi airfield 75, 78

Macaulay, Zachary and Kenneth 24
malaria 31, 39, 43, 46
Mapp Pharmaceuticals company 1
Massaquoi, Martha 82
Massumi, Brian 128
Mayor's Commission on African
  and Asian Heritage 'Delivering
  Shared heritage' report 135
Mbembe, Achille 9, 38, 59, 61, 62, 65,
  69, 79-80, 89
McKittrick, Katherine 123, 125, 140,
  147, 155
  Dear Science and Other Stories
  135-6
medevac *see* health care workers,
  evacuation of
medical expertise 123-4, 126, 144-8
  Black medical expertise 141, 144-7
  and whiteness 141, 146-51
medical humanitarianism 3-4
medical racism 10-12, 14, 17, 30,
  39-40, 51
Médicins Sans Frontières 1-2, 4, 98

miasma theory 45-6
Mignolo, Walter 15, 100-1
mobile ontologies 59, 61, 84-5,
  88-90, 161n2
  see also Black mobile ontologies
mobilities 58-90
  see also aeromobility; colonial
  mobilities; postcolonial mobilities
Mol, A. 94, 102, 104, 108, 118
Morrison, Toni *Beloved* 22-3
Mukwende, Malone [et al.] *Mind the
  Gap* 11

Nading, Alex 7
National Archives, Kew 26
neo-colonialism 128-9, 130-1, 133-4
New York, transport links to London
  62
New York Times 2-3
Nigeria 68, 76
Nigeria Airways 77
Noxolo, Patricia 60

O'Hare, Bernadette 129
Obama, Barack 132
Olufemi, Lola v
  Experiments in Imagining Otherwise
  157-8
ontopolitics 94
Operation 'Weary' 75
Owens, Deirdre Cooper 12

Pademba Road Cemetery, Waterloo
  xv-xix, xvii*ill*, xviii*ill*
Patterson, Orlando 9
people of colour 10, 16, 114, 127, 129
personal protective equipment (PPP)
  50-1, 113
Peters, Thomas 26
Philip, M. NourbeSe *Zong!* 71-3
phrenology 12
Pickens, Theri Alice 96
Piepzna-Samarasinha, Leah Lakshmi
  Care Work 92-3, 96, 99
Pierre, Jemima 9, 10, 16
Portuguese colonialism 22

postcolonial mobilities 61, 70–1, 89–90, 141, 146
postcolonial theory xix
Prescod-Weinstein, Chanda 124
Public Health Agency of Canada 1

race 4, 12–13, 44, 65, 100, 102–3, 125, 147, 155
    epigrammatic analysis of 155
racialisation 11, 16, 102, 104
racism 11, 13–14, 103, 136, 139–40, 157–8
    see also antiblackness; medical racism
Rankin, F. Harrison *The White Man's Grave* 17, 33–5, 45–6
RedR (volunteer organisation) 147, 149
Richards, Paul 124
Richardson, E.T. [et al.] 52, 100
Rogers, Tony 81
Ross, Ronald 30, 39, 43, 48, 161n8
Royal Air Maroc 80, 87, 88
Royal Gazette (journal) 71
Royal Geographical Society (RGS) 17, 67
Royal Hospital and Asylum 33, 36, 37–8
Royal Society meeting on Ebola (2016) 126–33, 162n1
Rubyan-Ling, David 147, 154

St Edward's church, Kent 22
Samaritan's Purse (medical mission) 2, 3
Securiport company 162n12
Sepúlveda, Juan Ginés de 9
Sharpe, Christina xix, 22, 42, 73, 90, 95, 114
    In the Wake 8
Sharpe, Granville 24–5
Sheller, Mimi 59, 80
Sheppard, Eric 62, 71
shipping infrastructures 73
Sierra Leone 17
    burial customs in 53
    civil war (1991-2002) 20, 31

dependency on UK 76, 78–81, 88–90, 131, 134, 140, 146, 155
    independence from UK (1961) 20, 74, 76–7, 70, 82
    granting of tax concessions to UK 129
    mobility links with UK 59–67
Sierra Leone Airways 77
Sierra Leone Company 21, 24, 25–6, 70
Sierra Leone Peace and Cultural Monument 26–7
Sierra Leonean diaspora 20, 80–1, 83–7, 88–90, 147, 149, 151–4, 155
Silva, Denise Ferreira da 100, 102
Simone, Abdoumaliq 76
Sirleaf, Ellen Johnson 132
slave ships 43, 62–3
slavery and slave trade xvii, 5, 10, 19–23, 32–6, 62–3, 79–80, 133
    apprenticeships for freed slaves 36, 96–7
    enslaved women 34–5
social Darwinism 39
South Africa 76, 143–4
Spillers, Hortense 9
spirometers 12
Sprecher, Armand 2
Stevens, Siaka 97
Stoler, Ann 27, 38, 65, 79
Sub-Saharan Africa 5, 11, 16, 63, 146
Suzuki, Yuka 141, 146

Taylor, Logan 43, 46, 48
Temne people 27
Torchlight (newspaper) 81–2
transport infrastructures 73–4

UN Humanitarian Air Services 74
United States, and Liberia 132, 133

valium *see* diazepam
Valladolid Debate (1550-51) 9

wake work 20
Walcott, Rinaldo 9

weather 22–4, 42–3, 47–8, 49–51
  see also antiblackness
Weheliye, Alexander 9, 102–3, 104
  Habeas Viscus 4
West Africa 4, 17–18, 192, 23, 43, 48,
  60, 63
  and aeromobilities 68–9, 74, 76–8
  climate in 44, 46–7
West Africa (magazine) 68
West African Airways Corporation
  (WAAC) 68–9, 76
West African Medical Service
  (WAMS) 30, 48
Westminster Group plc 78
White, Luise 52, 55
white settlers 93, 133
Wilberforce, William 24
Wilberforce, Freetown 28

Wilberforce Street 25ill
Wilkinson, Moses 24, 25
World Food Programme (WFP) 74
World Health Organization (WHO)
  1, 3, 144
Wynter, Sylvia v, xix, 9, 15–16, 23,
  100–3, 124, 158

yellow fever 31, 39–40, 43–4, 46,
  141
Yellow Fever Report (1913) 66
Yusoff, Kathryn 14

Zimbabwe 141–2
ZMapp (drug) 1–4
Zong (slave ship) 71–3, 161n6
  enslaved thrown overboard from
  72–3

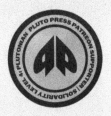

Thanks to our Patreon subscriber:

Ciaran Kane

Who has shown generosity and comradeship in support of our publishing.

Check out the other perks you get by subscribing to our Patreon – visit patreon.com/plutopress. Subscriptions start from £3 a month.

The Pluto Press Newsletter

Hello friend of Pluto!

Want to stay on top of the best radical books
we publish?

Then sign up to be the first to hear about our
new books, as well as special events,
podcasts and videos.

You'll also get 50% off your first order with us
when you sign up.

Come and join us!

Go to bit.ly/PlutoNewsletter